The Management of Procedure-Induced Anxiety in Children

T0201411

'Educational and enlightening, this book is like turning a light on with regards to how children feel and behave when they get anxious and stressed. All healthcare professionals will find it incredibly useful for understanding how children actually feel and their response to fear caused by the need for any sort of medical intervention, and how this can develop over time to become a major phobia. Not only does this book teach us about behaviour, it also shows us how we can modify and change what we do and how we do it to positively influence the children we look after and care for. The techniques and strategies described made me reconsider and change how I behave when I come across children in a healthcare setting, and how I behave with my own (young) children. This is rare in a "textbook", but then this is not a regular textbook, and I would urge anyone working with children throughout healthcare to read and treasure it.'

Dr Andrew Klein
Consultant, Royal Papworth Hospital, Cambridge, UK
Editor-in-Chief, *Anaesthesia*
Macintosh Professor, Royal College of Anaesthetists, London, UK, 2019

'*The Management of Procedure-Induced Anxiety in Children* by Richard Martin is one of the most interesting factual books I have read for a very long time.

Richard Martin shows that recognition by the operative team (including anaesthesiologists, surgeons, nurses and operating room staff and technicians) makes an enormous difference not only to the child's experience before, during and immediately after surgery, but also in the weeks following surgery.

There is so much that I could say about this book, but I think that it is summed up beautifully by a subheading that is labelled "we all communicate". This book demonstrates that communication is the key to both understanding and improving a child's procedure-induced anxiety.

I think that this book should be part of the core curriculum for doctors or other providers in anaesthesia, surgery and nursing. It is easy to read and evidence based. In years to come, it will be considered a game-changer with respect to how healthcare providers view and understand procedure-induced anxiety in children.'

Ken K. Nischal MD, FAAP, FRCOphth
Division Chief, Pediatric Ophthalmology and Strabismus
Medical Director, Digital Medicine, UPMC Children's Hospital of Pittsburgh
Professor, University of Pittsburgh, School of Medicine

The Management of Procedure-Induced Anxiety in Children

Dr Richard Martin
Great Ormond Street Hospital

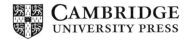
CAMBRIDGE
UNIVERSITY PRESS

CAMBRIDGE
UNIVERSITY PRESS

University Printing House, Cambridge CB2 8BS, United Kingdom

One Liberty Plaza, 20th Floor, New York, NY 10006, USA

477 Williamstown Road, Port Melbourne, VIC 3207, Australia

314–321, 3rd Floor, Plot 3, Splendor Forum, Jasola District Centre, New Delhi – 110025, India

79 Anson Road, #06–04/06, Singapore 079906

Cambridge University Press is part of the University of Cambridge.

It furthers the University's mission by disseminating knowledge in the pursuit of education, learning, and research at the highest international levels of excellence.

www.cambridge.org
Information on this title: www.cambridge.org/9781108822947
DOI: 10.1017/9781108913317

First published 2021

Printed in the United Kingdom by TJ Books Limited, Padstow Cornwall

A catalogue record for this publication is available from the British Library.

Library of Congress Cataloging-in-Publication Data
Names: Martin, Richard (Consultant Paediatric
    Anaesthetist), author.
Title: The management of procedure-induced anxiety in children /
    Richard Martin.
Description: New York, NY : Cambridge University Press, 2021. |
    Includes bibliographical references and index.
Identifiers: LCCN 2020055287 (print) | LCCN 2020055288 (ebook)
    | ISBN 9781108822947 (paperback) | ISBN 9781108913317 (epub)
Subjects: MESH: Surgical Procedures, Operative–psychology | Child |
    Anxiety–prevention & control | Professional-Patient Relations
Classification: LCC RD32 (print) | LCC RD32 (ebook) |
    NLM WO 925 | DDC 617.9–dc23
LC record available at https://lccn.loc.gov/2020055287
LC ebook record available at https://lccn.loc.gov/2020055288

ISBN 978-1-108-82294-7 Paperback

Contents

Preface

Helping to support anxious children in medical practice has been my passion since the late 1990s. From then until now, I have been lucky enough to be on this journey: a journey of evolution for both the subject and myself. During this time, I have come to understand what I believe are the considerations that are fundamental to the success of any initiative to address the mental health of children who experience procedure-induced anxiety. In my humble opinion, these considerations are as follows:

- Children experiencing procedure-induced anxiety are best served by the many, armed with a core competency to do so
- The training required to support such activity must be embraced and delivered by our governing institutions
- While the day-to-day management of these children should be delivered predominantly by these many, there will be children with more significant and challenging issues that will require the support of a multidisciplinary group with advanced training in this field of practice
- Finally, but most important of all, this initiative and the understanding that will dictate training and practice belongs to every single one of us. It does not belong to, and should not be delivered by, any single individual or subgroup of individuals. The nature of any solution and evaluation of subject material must be inclusive, collaborative – never exclusive. We know only what we know, never what we don't know – yet others may

With this in mind, you would be justified in asking why I have written this textbook as a single author, and you would not be alone. I asked myself the very same question. In answer to this, first, I wished to share everything and anything I knew or had thought on this subject, with a view to connecting with others who were similarly inquisitive, in the hope they may be encouraged to take up the baton and run with it. Second, I believe this text merely contributes momentum to just the *beginning* of a far, far greater and incredibly exciting dialogue and exchange of ideas that is yet to come. I believe the time is right.

I feel incredibly privileged to have stumbled upon this area of interest. It represents a home and outlet to who I am and what I feel passionate about. I hope this is reflected in the practices, ideas and perspectives I have tried to represent in this book and I hope this will encourage and inspire you to begin or continue the invaluable journey of your own. Everything you do makes a difference.

Acknowledgements

My journey to this point would never have started without the support of my mother. She instilled in me the belief that everything and anything is possible, while securing an environment rich with opportunity. As a teacher with a degree in psychology, I watched her utilise behaviour management strategies and listened to her explain the origins and complexities of these techniques. As such, she was the first to fan the flames of an interest in people and behaviour that has led me to this point. I feel compelled to additionally acknowledge the outstanding training in hypnotherapy I was lucky enough to receive, as well as the eternal positive support and ongoing friendship from Gavin Emerson. His influence came at a critical time in my journey leading to a fundamental shift in direction both professionally and personally. Leaving the most important of all to last, I would not miss an opportunity to thank Clare, my wife. She has patiently supported me throughout my journey, no matter where it has taken me. She is my best friend, my wife and an exceptional mother to our four children. She and my family will always be, hands down, the most important thing to me in life. Without Clare's support and encouragement, I would not have been able to write this book. She must take equal credit for the completion of this book and any improvement in the experiences of children it may encourage.

Introduction

1.1 Terminology

Procedure-Induced Anxiety (PIA)

By definition **Procedure-Induced Anxiety (PIA)** is anxiety that is induced by any procedure whether in anticipation of this procedure or as the direct consequence of the experience at the time.

Operative Procedure-Induced Anxiety (OPIA)

Referring to PIA as opposed to peri-operative anxiety is intentional. Perioperative anxiety, by definition, references anxiety associated with operative procedures, and excludes that experienced by the numerically superior non-operative medical procedure group. As such, it is not an overarching term. With a view to seeking such overarching, definitive terminology, perioperative anxiety can be redefined as **Operative Procedure-Induced Anxiety (OPIA)** which would represent a subgroup of children within the overarching group who experience PIA.

Procedure-Induced Psychological Trauma (PIPT)

Procedure-Induced Psychological Trauma is the psychological morbidity experienced as a direct consequence of PIA.

Post-procedure Dysfunctional Behaviour (PPDB)

Post-procedure Dysfunctional Behaviour is defined as new, dysfunctional behaviour that develops as a direct consequence of PIPT.

Post-operative Dysfunctional Behaviour (PODB)

As with the terms PIA and OPIA, **Post-operative Dysfunctional Behavior (PODB)** is a subset of PPDB in that it only references new dysfunctional behaviour, manifested as a direct consequence of operative interventions.

1.2 Anxiety, Fear and Fight/Flight

It is understandable, even to be expected, that a child attending hospital for a medical procedure will experience some degree of anxiety. Anxiety in and of itself is a natural response. It is the physical and psychological manifestation of the body's preparation to defend itself against an unknown threat. Research suggests that the response to a *known* threat is different, evolving via a different pathway in the brain and manifests as fear.

It is worth noting that individuals with high trait anxiety, revealed on testing using the STAIC questionnaire (State-Trait Anxiety Inventory for Children – Spielberger) (1), show early activation of the neurophysiological pathway involved in the generation of anxiety (2).

While unpleasant or uncomfortable, the sensation of feeling anxious does not cause further harm unless it is allowed to grow unchecked in the presence of continued anxiogenic stimuli. This can happen if the child has no coping strategies or the stimulation increases due to inappropriate handling or mismanagement by the family or medical team. If the anxiety continues to go unchecked, it may evolve further into a full-blown fight or flight response.

Some children experience such extreme anxiety and fear that they develop a phobic patterned response to medical interventions and all stimuli associated with them. If an anxious and reluctant child is forced to comply so that a medical procedure can take place, it can be terrifying, making development of phobic responses more likely. The experience of being terrified yet being forced to comply by grown adults can cause such psychological trauma that a fear of fear itself can evolve and persist long after any fear of medical interventions has resolved.

With regards to the fight–flight response that we are so familiar with from the literature, we should note that calling it a fight–flight response is incorrect. Generally what one will see is best described as a freeze–flight–fight response. The first action will be to become noticeably still and attempt to avoid attention by adopting a body position that may make you physically smaller or involve turning away to avoid engagement. If this fails, the option may be taken to move away or even run and hide. A last resort, if all else has failed, will be to offer physical resistance, to fight (3).

In a perfect world, all clinicians would be trained to minimise and effectively manage anxiety. There should be a screening system in place to detect those at greatest risk of experiencing this emotion with a view to preventive intervention.

On a more positive note, a child can develop a phobic state through conditioning, yet this same process can help any child move in the opposite direction, towards a more positive state, albeit with time, patience and appropriate support.

1.2.1 Nature of the Anxiety State

The state is dominated by a ramping of anxiety towards fear, with a parallel ramping of the physiological changes encountered when the freeze–flight–fight response is triggered. The triggering of the pituitary adrenal axis and release of catecholamines is responsible for many of the physical and psychological consequences that we are all familiar with. But as adults our appraisal of the experience we gain from such an event will be very different to that of a child, particularly children under 5 years of age.

As medical professionals you will be aware of the effects of adrenaline and noradrenaline on the body. A child will experience all of these including the racing heart, tachypnoea, dry mouth and stasis of the gastrointestinal system with associated nausea. Those most severely affected may feel the need to defaecate or micturate. Experiencing these physical changes, the sense of losing control and the disruption of a child's familiar and predictable existence with the disorientation that brings can be understandably terrifying.

From any physician's perspective, it is distressing to experience a child so severely affected that you can feel them sweating, the heat they are generating and their heart pounding through the T-shirt they are wearing as you rest a supportive hand on their shoulder. You may see them hyperventilating and attempting to shrink from sight by moving towards their best approximation of the foetal position. They may even soil themselves if their distress is not noted and appropriately managed. In this situation, anything less than diffusing the situation by generating space and releasing the pressure will at best reinforce the conditioned response and at worst further severely traumatise the child.

Additional changes we will be unaware of in this situation are sensory changes experienced by the child. Changes in the field of vision and auditory sensitivities may vary from child to child. Needless to say, they will be in a state of hypervigilance. From a cognitive perspective they may find it difficult to understand more complex communication and abstract concepts. You may find that, in order to help them extract themselves from this extreme state, you need to connect utilising highly simplified forms of verbal communication and, as they emerge from the fog associated with this state, you can move slowly towards more age-appropriate and complex forms of dialogue.

Of particular note, we should draw attention to the fact that this anxiety state is characterised by an *internal focus* with *internal dialogue*, the subject and content of which are dictated by the state itself. They will be squarely focused on how awful this experience is for them and how it makes them feel. This focus and dialogue represents a further barrier to any individual attempting to manage the anxiety or help them manage it themselves. In order to implement any successful strategy, you will first need to reach the child and, in so doing, move them from an internally focused state with their own internal dialogue, towards an externally focused state, fully engaged with some external stimulus and distracted from any internal monologue. Techniques specifically designed to achieve this are described and highlighted as such in later sections.

There is new evidence relating to the freeze–flight–fight response and fear. Some researchers have discovered that catecholamines have a profound effect in the amygdala. We know that memories associated with fear tend to be very powerful and vivid. It is thought that catecholamines released during frightening experiences augment memory formation making them more vivid and longer lasting (4–6).

Understanding this process further informs us with regards to the development of anxiety states and PTSD. Additionally, this significantly contributes to our appreciation of conditioned phobic response following extreme anxiogenic stimuli and the realities of children experiencing PIA, PIPT and the consequential morbidity (6).

1.2.2 Threat until Proven Otherwise and Overwhelming Message: Non-threat

It is important to grasp that the process we are referring to and the behavioural pattern we see as a consequence have positive survival benefits. They are core primitive responses, coded deep into the essence of who and what we are. Unsurprisingly, activation of this process is significantly influenced by past negative experience and patterned response can evolve following repetitive exposure. In the presence of such conditioning, individuals that are affected in this way will likely treat any and every stimulus within their vicinity as a threat until unequivocally proven otherwise.

With this in mind, we can appreciate a core principle in the management of PIA – that the goal of any management strategy is to broadcast an *overwhelming message of non-threat*. This is achieved by utilising a mixture of effective strategies that contribute to an overwhelming and congruent message of non-threat, that is communicated continuously until hypervigilance is brought under control, trust is established and an alternate narrative incorporating an effective coping strategy is implemented.

1.3 Why Some Children Manage Their Anxiety and Others Don't

The ability to manage anxiety hinges on two factors. The first factor is the anxiogenic load the child is exposed to. No matter how able or capable a child might be, there is a limit to any individual's capacity to cope. In the presence of an anxiogenic stimulus of sufficient magnitude, all children will fail to manage their PIA. Within the realms of normal hospital practice, the vast majority of interventions, if not all, can be managed clinically and psychologically in such a way that PIA and further PIPT is minimised. In the presence of significant PIPT, to achieve such a positive outcome it may be imperative that elective therapy is undertaken to address such trauma before further medical interventions can proceed. If this does not happen, the child is likely to sustain additional PIPT as a consequence. The second factor is the child's possession and ability to deploy effective coping strategies.

1.3.1 Coping Strategies

What are they? They are:

> constantly changing cognitive and behavioural efforts to manage specific external and/or internal demands that are appraised as taxing or exceeding the resources of the person.
>
> (R. S. Lazarus & S. Folkman, *Stress Appraisal and Coping*, Springer, 1984)

Essentially, coping strategies are a means to cope with a stressful situation or anxiogenic stimulus.

In the absence of these, minimally stressful or anxiogenic stimuli can very quickly overwhelm a child. Additionally, coping strategies may, for whatever reason, be present but inaccessible leading to a similar negative outcome. Lastly, we must accept that any coping strategy, no matter how effective, will not maintain the status quo indefinitely. If the stimulus is of sufficient magnitude or longevity, any strategy will eventually be overwhelmed.

Coping strategies fall into one of two broad categories. They either allow the child to alter their perspective or evaluation of the situation, or they allow them to focus on something else, often by accessing positive resources (discussed in Section 1.4).

Examples of techniques allowing re-evaluation of any threat would include a cognitive approach such as establishing in one's own mind that although the situation is unpleasant, there is value in accepting what needs to be done in order to get better. Similarly, fixating on a future positive outcome as a result of the intervention, such as following some type of plastic surgery that will significantly alter the child's appearance in a positive way, would have a similar effect. One last example would be to highlight what we see in far too many children who have had multiple negative experiences from an early age over a long period of time and have been negatively conditioned. If we manage to intervene in a manner that changes this experience in a way that it becomes manageable and less unpleasant, it is possible for them to relearn and be reconditioned. In such a situation, they may still have an overwhelming conditioned drive for self-preservation in any medical environment, but if the process of rebuilding has begun in association with new, more positive experiences, they may be able to counter any negative internal dialogue by fixating on more recent positive experiences and challenge any negative thoughts that arise. Again, this is a cognitive approach.

Internal distraction techniques that allow a child to focus on something more positive such as memories or experiences linked to positive emotions is another form of coping strategy. The ability for such an approach to achieve the desired effect will inevitably depend on the child's ability to manage such an approach effectively. This type of strategy has been noted as developing in older patient groups and is an abstraction of reality only possible at more advanced stages of cognitive development. Younger children are less likely to be able to use such techniques. A positive outcome in this situation hinges on the balance between the negative stimulus and the positive strategy. There are many techniques mentioned in later sections that utilise this type of approach. In fact, it is probably the most common core strategy. Examples include guided imagery, whether formally taught or deployed as the consequence of natural aptitude, humour and formal distraction. And there are many others. The presence or absence of strategies is influenced by cognitive development, personality traits, family and past experience.

In terms of cognitive development, the age group most likely to struggle with procedure-induced anxiety (PIA) are children who are 5 years old and under. Within this group, the ability to understand the reasons for intervention, the sense of self and the ability to construct associations and understanding of a more complex nature are limited. As a result, the ability to develop and deploy coping strategies is limited. Naturally, the presence of learning difficulties and the associated impairment of cognitive function may result in similar difficulties in older children.

The child's personality traits inevitably influence their outlook and the nature of the process leading to formulating coping strategies. With the advent of Spielberger's State Trait Anxiety Inventory (STAI), there followed a multitude of research papers describing the traits associated with an increased vulnerability in terms of PIA. Historically, these traits have been defined as high emotionality combined with low sociability, which translate to highly emotional or more emotional children who are less socially capable or more introverted. As noted above, those with these traits tend to show early activation of the neural pathway whose function is the signalling of anxiety, in comparison to children without these traits. Why one child develops this pattern of personality traits as opposed to another is complex and multifactorial. It may depend on genetics, conditioning, family structure, relationships within the family and physical interaction with the environment.

The influence of family relationships and structure is unsurprising. For anyone working with children, the influence stressed or anxious parents have upon their children will be very familiar. The family environment will dictate a child's expectations of life and their behaviour. They will learn what to do from parents and siblings, and they will utilise modelling behaviour by observing their family members in different situations and copying them. If parents or siblings are themselves anxious by nature, then this will significantly influence the nature of others in the unit. Lastly, there may be negative influences at play within the unit in the form of a situation where negative behaviour including dependence and emotional dysfunction are actually encouraged. This is often due to actual or perceived secondary gain experienced by other family members. This influence can be transgenerational, as its aetiology may be from the grandparents or beyond, and the aetiology of such behaviour may be negative past medical experience on behalf of the perpetrator.

Past experiences can significantly affect a child's ability to cope. If a child has had positive experiences when undergoing medical interventions, this can act as a resource for them and is likely to positively influence their outlook and response to subsequent interventions. Naturally, not all experiences are guaranteed to be pleasant, yet an unpleasant experience managed effectively may act as a positive resource, bolster a child's confidence and help them manage challenging situations in the future.

In truth, there are many significant ingredients that contribute to a positive experience, from clinical effectiveness to psychological elements such as being told the truth – not being lied to. Even in the presence of significant negative past experiences, a well-thought-out, effective management plan can begin the process of repairing damage done to a child as the consequence of poorly managed PIA.

Children who have experienced poorly managed PIA from an early age and on multiple occasions will not only have difficulty coping with any medical interventions, they are also likely to develop a phobic response to all aspects of hospital care, including sensory stimuli that have never been associated with anxiogenic stimuli. Simply attending the hospital can be enough to precipitate a panic attack, autonomic activation or a full-blown freeze–flight–fight response. This illustrates the manner in which severe anxiety can evolve and manifest as a malignant, invasive psychological condition. Those who have worked with children experiencing this type of difficulty will recognise this description and may accept the term 'global malignant anxiety disorder' as an overarching term. For some children, the anxiety they may experience as a consequence of hospital care can lead to anxiety spreading and invading other, unrelated aspects of their daily existence. These individuals require specialist multidisciplinary support and interventions if a more balanced existence is to be re-established.

Those looking for an excellent and comprehensive account of research in this subject area should read the work of Rudolph et al. (1995) (7).

1.4 Resources

What are they?

Resources fall within two broad categories. First is information that aids in rapport building. Examples would include the child's favourite things, their hobbies, songs they like, if they have any pets, if they have brothers or sisters and any other interests they might have. Such information will inform conversation that will interest and engage the child, while at the same time allowing the other participant in the conversation to interact with them on a more intimate level; in essence, building rapport or an equity between child and clinician. We will discuss rapport in more detail in Section 1.5.

The second category includes a child's memories, experiences and interests that are associated with positive memories, conditioned behaviour and emotions. Memories stored in context, based upon an experience and of any nature, positive or negative in valence, were described by Tulving as episodic memories – memories that include context and on retrieval of which the individual will relive the experience in all associated aspects and in its original context. This will inevitably include reliving the emotional content of such memories (8, 9).

Knowledge of this type of memory or the ability to access a stereotypically predictable memory by referring to it in broad and general terms, such as asking the child to remember their favourite place in the whole world, will aid in management of PIA by helping the child relive a positive experience and therefore any associated emotions, rather than focusing on the negative ones they may be currently struggling to deal with. In truth, there is no need to know specifics with regards to a child's memories or experiences. Even when a child offers no details of such experiences, simply asking them to remember or access something that made them feel happy and safe or made them laugh, in association with other supportive measures, may be enough to help them access positive resources, emotions and a more positive emotional state.

An understanding of this type of resource offers a clinician the means to shift the focus of attention in any interaction, away from a challenging and potentially negative clinical situation, towards the positive memories, emotions, feelings and behaviour encapsulated within the episodic memory. This represents a powerful coping strategy that can be deployed instantly by any attending clinician with a view to helping any child struggling to manage PIA.

1.5 Operative Procedure-Induced Anxiety (OPIA)

The majority of children admitted to hospital will experience anxiety. The risk of experiencing anxiety will inevitably increase if a child undergoes some form of intervention.

From the anaesthetists' perspective, we will mainly be interested in research defining perioperative anxiety, but should appreciate that anxiety associated with intervention is not unique to anaesthesia and surgery. It occurs as a consequence of any medical intervention.

There is a wealth of published research defining perioperative anxiety, its prevalence and consequences. In exploring this data, as anaesthetists examining the association between anxiety, anxiety at induction of anaesthesia and the consequent morbidity, it is important to acknowledge that the anaesthetic or surgery itself are not causative. The psychological trauma and morbidity that we see in children after an intervention is the consequence of the anxiety and fear these children experience. Any new post-hospital or post-intervention dysfunctional behaviour seen in these children is an outward manifestation of this trauma.

1.5.1 Incidence of OPIA

The prevalence of OPIA can vary significantly from study to study. One recent study stated the number of children experiencing anxiety during their intervention was in the nineties, percentage wise. A more consistent median range, taken from studies within a suitably extensive timeframe, would suggest 40–60% prevalence would be more accurate (10). Therefore, it may be that the majority of children under our care suffer from anxiety.

1.5.2 Consequences of OPIA

Anxiety in and of itself is unpleasant. If it is not managed effectively, if it intensifies to a point where the child cannot cope, if it evolves into fear or terror, or it triggers a freeze–flight–fight response, then the child is likely to sustain some degree of Procedure-Induced Psychological Trauma or PIPT as a consequence. This may manifest itself in a number of different ways and for a variable time following surgery. The most extensively studied and reported manifestation is in the form of Postoperative Dysfunctional Behaviour – PODB. These patterns of behaviour can be seen on a short-term and long-term basis. There is some research that prompts the question as to whether early childhood psychological trauma might be linked to life-long consequences and even a reduced lifespan.

1.5.3 Short-Term

Short-term dysfunctional behaviour generally refers to new dysfunctional behaviour seen within the first 3 weeks to 3 months following any intervention. Research published throughout the last century, reports a prevalence of PODB between 24 and 60% of children within the initial post-intervention period (11–15).

These new behaviours resolve quickly in the majority of children. However, in some these patterns of dysfunction will persist into the medium and long-term post-intervention period. It goes without saying that this is both disturbing for the child and their parents.

The list below is not exhaustive but illustrative, and includes patterns reported in the literature over the last 100 years.

- Regression of developmental milestones – for example returning to requiring nappies
- Bed wetting
- Nightmares or night terrors
- Problems sleeping
- Problems with eating
- Separation anxiety
- Temper tantrums
- Problems with authority
- Fear of strangers or the dark
- Fear of the unfamiliar
- Fear of doctors and procedures or pain
- Fear of being lied to
- Fear of being held down

Three generic papers that grant an overview of the extensive body of research from this period are referenced here (16–18).

1.5.4 Long-Term

For some children, these patterns of behaviour persist. Between 4 and 12% of children continue to display new dysfunctional behaviour for more than a year following surgery (15, 19). Undoubtedly, if there are multiple interventions that precipitate fear and extreme anxiety over a period of time, the consequences are likely to be significant and long-lasting. Examples of the types of behaviour that may be seen are included in the list below. Again, this list is illustrative.

- Low self-esteem
- Anxiety neuroses
- Global malignant anxiety – a generalised progressive invasive anxiety
- Eating disorders
- Phobias
- Depression
- Immune suppression
- PTSD

1.5.5 Life-Long?

There is a growing body of evidence that adverse childhood events and experiences are linked to compromise in mental health in later life. Patterns of behaviour that have been linked to childhood trauma include depression, alcohol dependence, self-harm, suicide, drug abuse, conduct disorder and violence. Of particular note, childhood trauma is clearly linked to PTSD (20, 21).

One landmark research project conducted by Vincent Felitti and his team was published in 1998 (22). The Adverse Childhood Experiences (ACE) study looked at the impact of adverse childhood events or ACEs on both mental and physical health in adult life. This study unsurprisingly illustrated an incremental relationship between the number of adverse childhood events experienced and the risk of developing mental health illness in later life. What was surprising to some degree was that the study also revealed an incremental relationship between the number of ACEs experienced and lifestyle choices that were linked to physical illnesses such as heart disease, diabetes and chronic lung disease. As such, this research made a connection between psychological trauma in childhood and lifestyle choices that were directly linked to physical illness in later life and a reduction in life expectancy. Additional evidence supporting an association between negative experiences in childhood, morbidity and reduced lifespan has continued to emerge over the years since Felitti's work was first published. A recently published meta-analysis of research in this area of interest supports an association between certain types of early life adversity, the early onset of puberty, structural changes within the brain and reduced lifespan (23).

When we consider the impact of PIA and hospital admissions and in particular the experience of children undergoing multiple interventions associated with pain, anxiety and fear, it is impossible *not* to view these episodes as adverse childhood events. As such, does this not imply that exposure to such events will have consequences similar to those found in the research outlined above. Is PIA linked to long-term psychological and physical morbidity with a consequent reduction in lifespan?

1.5.6 Transgenerational

The transgenerational effect of PIA is commonly seen by clinicians working with children and their families. We have all met parents and grandparents with their own past negative experiences of healthcare and PIA. Many of them struggle with feelings and emotions precipitated either by the medical environment itself or witnessing the experiences of the child they are supporting through treatment. These emotions and feelings are stored with their own episodic memories from the past and surface as a type of negative resource (8). When these emotions surface, the parents' or grandparents' behaviour may become maladaptive as they struggle with their feelings and memories of the anxiety and fear they experienced themselves. If this happens, they may offer commentary on the current situation and by sharing their own past negative experiences, they may negatively influence the child they are attempting to support. It is worth noting, although this might make both the child's situation more difficult for them to manage and our management of the situation more of a challenge, it does not represent a deliberate act of sabotage. Additionally, we must acknowledge that the successful management of a child's anxiety will inevitably require the management of anxiety experienced by any influential member of their family.

1.6 Post-operative Dysfunctional Behaviour: UK Statistics

To illustrate the significance of PIA, research statistics have been used to project actual numbers of children affected in The UK each year. Data published by The Office For National Statistics and NHS Digital are used to assist in this goal.

Population UK < 18y (House of Commons Report 2016)	13,881,000 (24)	
NHS Digital – Hospital Episodes Statistics 2017–18 Admitted patient procedures < 18y	100%	784,814
Children experiencing anxiety at induction of anaesthesia	40–60%	313,925–470,888
Children displaying PODB 3w after surgery	24–60%	188,355–470,888
Children displaying PODB 1y after surgery	4–12%	31,392–94,177

To put these figures into context, if you accept that on average around 8% of children undergoing surgery still display PODB one full year after the intervention, the number of children affected in one year represents approximately 0.5% of the UK population under the age of 18.

1.7 Critical Elements of Child–Clinician Interaction

1.7.1 Rapport

A close and harmonious relationship in which the people or groups concerned understand each other's feelings or ideas and communicate well.

Oxford English Dictionary

We are all aware of rapport to some extent, with some of us more sensitive to it than others. How to build rapport in a positive manner will be discussed later as part of the management strategy section (Section 1.3.1). For now, it is enough to draw attention to its importance in the anxiety management process and caution against damaging rapport. At the core of the definition above, is the implication that the central element in rapport is a connection underpinned by attentiveness and an intention to reach an understanding. People respond positively to those they feel they have a rapport with and equally negatively to those with whom rapport is damaged or completely lost.

It is unfortunate that rapport can so easily be lost. A clinician's role serves both purpose and process, with the purpose being to care for the patient in body and mind. The process inevitably involves sifting through information garnered by posing a network of questions, designed to reach a medical diagnosis, and requiring careful documentation. Such a process can easily dominate any interaction, particularly for the inexperienced or functionally overloaded practitioner. The result can be that this process obscures and undermines rapport building by preventing the formation of a therapeutic connection between patient and clinician.

1.7.2 Trust

Trust is of paramount importance as a core principle in the management of PIA. Children rely on parents and adults to ensure their safety, wellbeing and stability in their lives. With this in mind they trust their parents or adult guardians. From an evolutionary perspective there is a positive survival benefit in this, as a vulnerable child will depend upon adults for everything. With this in mind, medical interventions present an issue for some family units. For some adults, informing their child that they will be having a possibly painful and distressing intervention represents a task well outside their experience and absent from their skillset as a parent. Under these circumstances it is understandable that they may determine that *not* telling their child what is going to happen is the best option. They may even be of the opinion their child is incapable of understanding and it is in their best interests not to know the truth. Irrespective of the parents' ability or the child's capacity to understand, this is undoubtedly a mistake. If a child is not informed or is lied to, their belief that the adults caring for them will ensure their safety and the integrity of their existence is challenged if not permanently undermined. As a direct consequence, their main source of support and reassurance at a time of maximal vulnerability will have been removed. Not only can this in itself lead to significant anxiety and psychological trauma but also fear and panic. The effects and consequences of damage to the trust between child and parent can extend well after the traumatising event. If this occurs, the parent will have removed themselves as the prime resource for reassurance and support in the post-intervention period. If such a sequence of events occurs on more than one occasion and over time, the damage may be irreparable.

This situation is all too familiar for any clinician working with children and it is a scenario that is as old as time itself as evidenced by Eckenhoff in 1953 (17). In this paper he describes two cases where a negative outcome is the result of a child being lied to. In 1945, Levy commented on prophylactic measures to minimise the trauma of medical interventions. He clearly states that children should receive a simple yet clear explanation of what they can expect to happen (16).

So, we should aim to inform children under our care. We should educate parents with regards to the benefits of honesty and the pitfalls of lying to their child. For those parents who are struggling with this or feel their child will not cope we, as their clinicians, must be able to support the family unit in educating them and brokering a solution.

1.7.3 Compassion

Compassion, empathy and sympathy are integral to supportive behaviour patterns deployed by parents or indeed any human being towards another. Defined in the Cambridge English dictionary as:

> A strong feeling of sympathy and sadness for other people's suffering or bad luck and a desire to help.

Compassion is an important vehicle for offering support and signalling an outward confirmation that another individual's reality has been both noticed and understood. This is a form of validation which is discussed in more detail as a management strategy (Section 1.3.1). In the context of supporting a child through a difficult, challenging or unpleasant experience, the expression of compassion has great value. For the child it confirms their sources of support and security are still in place and it strengthens the positive emotional connection between parent and child. Similarly, compassion expressed by a clinician 'piggy-backs' upon this aspect of family interaction. By doing so, not only will this support the child, but the action significantly contributes to the rapport building process.

An absence of compassion does not simply leave a void, it makes a strong statement. It evidences a lack of compassion and implies one of three things. These are a lack of awareness, the view compassion is not warranted, or a decision not to offer compassion. With this in mind, the merits of compassion and the damage its absence can cause are easy to comprehend.

1.7.4 Compliance/Coercion

There is a sense of passivity to the word compliance. In recognising this, it should be clear that successful management of PIA is not about merely gaining compliance, it involves empowering children to manage their own anxiety whenever possible. If this is not achievable, we may be in a position where we must offer the child a ready-made coping strategy or deploy one on their behalf. Ultimately, however, the gold-standard should be autonomy. To attain this a child may require elective input from a specialist multidisciplinary team.

In addition to an understanding of compliance and autonomy, we should appreciate the potentially negative influence of coercion. It is possible to gain compliance by overwhelming a child through coercion. If this approach is taken intentionally or not, it can result in a further increase in the child's anxiety, fear of the individual who is coercing them and or anxiety and fear that someone else may seek to gain compliance by overwhelming their defences whenever they return for further interventions. Adults who are coerced tend to be left with a sense of being forced to do something they didn't really want to do (25, 26). This tends to result in resentment. In children one would guess this approach may be experienced as a psychological equivalent to gaining compliance by physical enforcement.

1.7.5 Restraint

It is difficult to imagine what it must be like to feel so anxious and frightened that you develop a freeze–flight–fight response, whereupon one or more adults physically restrain you, forcing you to tolerate whatever it was that you were terrified of in the first place. In contemplating this, we can understand why some children develop a fear of fear itself, simply a fear of being restrained and feeling terrified again, while concern over any intervention may have dwindled.

Restraint in response to anxiety and non-compliance is guaranteed to make a child's anxiety worse (27). As such and accepting there is a direct association between OPIA and psychological trauma manifesting as PODB (11), no clinician would advocate restraining a child in order to force compliance unless it was an absolute last resort, the intervention had to take place and there was no alternative (28).

Most institutions will have a policy document with a guide to the management of restraint for staff. In developing such a document, most institutions will reference a publication produced on behalf of The Royal College of Nursing (29). Most guidelines will outline the need for training in safe restraint, adequate numbers of staff to safely apply this approach, and a need for consent in advance and debriefing afterwards. They will also include clear commentary on the circumstances under which restraint can be acceptably implemented. Despite such policy documents, they are rarely if ever applied to the restraint utilised during anaesthetic induction. The reason for this is unclear and worthy of discussion.

Lastly, it is worth noting that there is a difference between restraint and, for example, confining a 2-year-old to the lap area of a parent. The former requires significant force that can itself add to the anxiogenic load the child is exposed to. If a child is distressed as the consequence of a medical intervention, being forced to comply in a potentially uncomfortable or even painful manner can only add to the confusion, emotional trauma and physical discomfort.

This latter point should be highlighted and appraised by clinicians with a view to establishing the merits of utilising a parent to deploy restraint. Many appear to see this as somehow preferable, or more ethically acceptable. However, when one considers the additional anxiogenic load restraint imposes on the child and the impact deploying restraint is likely to have upon trust and a parent's ability to credibly act as a supportive resource, one might argue the parent is the last person one might allow to restrain a child.

Key Points

- All children experience anxiety when exposed to unfamiliar surroundings, people and procedures.
- If anxiety levels go unchecked or reach a maximal level, a full freeze–flight–fight response may be triggered.
- Repeated exposure to such stimuli may result in a conditioned phobic response.
- A child's capacity to cope with anxiety is dictated by anxiogenic load balanced against their ability to deploy established coping strategies.
- The presence or absence of strategies is influenced by cognitive development, personality trait, family and past experience.
- Procedure-Induced Anxiety (PIA) is associated with significant Procedure-Induced Psychological Trauma (PIPT) that may manifest as Post-Procedure Dysfunctional Behaviour (PPDB).
- Naturally, Operative Procedure-Induced Anxiety (OPIA) and Post-Operative Dysfunctional Behaviour (PODB) are subgroups within PIA and PPDB respectively.
- Children don't just get over traumatic experiences – they *do* remember – and they remember for a long time.
- The effects of repeated negative experiences may last a lifetime.
- There is evidence that adverse childhood events or early life adversity, particularly experiencing or the perception of physical threat, may have a negative impact upon lifespan.
- Positive influences in the management of anxiety include rapport, trust and compassion.
- Aspects that have a negative impact upon anxiety management include coercion and restraint. It might be argued the use of coercion and or restraint represents a failure to implement optimal procedure-induced anxiety management.

Having established a foundation of understanding with regards to PIA, the next sections will outline advanced techniques that can be deployed as part of an effective management strategy aimed at reducing PIA and minimising consequent psychological morbidity.

Chapter

2

Emergent Management of Procedure-Induced Anxiety (PIA)

2.1 Core Principles

2.1.1 Altered State

When children are anxious, they are in an altered state. The altered state creates both opportunity and vulnerability by making a child more sensitive and responsive to both positive and negative comments or influences. What we say to them while in this state can have a profound effect upon them. We should therefore choose our words very carefully and proscriptively. Comments that can be perceived negatively can have a disproportionate influence.

2.1.2 Resistance

Anxious children are even more resistant to influence than children normally are. They will perceive everything as a threat until it is absolutely proven to be 'non-threat'. As a consequence, any attempt at reducing or managing anxiety will require the use of techniques that can be braided into normal patterns of behaviour in order to evade detection, appraisal and subsequent resistance. Additionally, the number and quality of non-threat stimuli will need to be of significant magnitude to overcome the child's drive for self-preservation.

2.1.3 Mass Effect

When we understand the nature of the anxiety state and the consequent drive for self-preservation, we can understand that it is rarely one element in effective communication or management that will deliver the desired outcome. It is the simultaneous covert deployment of a myriad of behaviours, subtleties of communication and coping strategies, all sending the same message, braided into an approach that appears to be nothing at all, that will achieve the desired endpoint.

2.1.4 Congruence

The issue of congruence with regards to the message we send is extremely important. All of the points of reference in our communication should send the same message. By ensuring this is achieved we will maximise the potential for a positive outcome. Any aspect of communication with an anxious child that is ambiguous or could be interpreted in a negative way could derail the process. A single negative can undermine multiple positives within the same interaction.

2.2 We All Communicate

We all communicate. A three-month-old baby will reciprocate a smile as at some level it recognises the positive survival benefit of such behaviour. Yes, there are some naturally good communicators among us for whom it is all intuitive, but we all communicate, every second of every day of our lives. Everyone, anyone can hone this skill if they want to. So, rather than good and bad communicators, there will be good and exceptional communicators. There is no excuse for poor communication unless there is impaired function due to pathology or behavioural dysfunction.

Chapter 3

Non-verbal Communication

Non-verbal communication, often referred to as body language, refers to the myriad of cues and signals we send and receive each and every moment, every day of our lives. A three-month-old baby will reciprocate a smile as the process of communicating begins the moment we are born and our mastery of interpretation and composition grows exponentially over time. As such, we are all experts in communication. It is agreed that some of us are exquisitely sensitive, the majority are at very least aware and competent, while a minority, often due to specific impairments, can struggle. With this in mind, what follows in this section is an appraisal of non-verbal communication, the work that has been carried out to help us understand how we interact, and the signalling, interpretation and dynamic interaction that might help us in managing procedure-induced anxiety (PIA). Aspects of non-verbal communication appraised in this section include the following:

- Proxemics
- Height
- Eye contact
- Facial expression
- Head movement
- Posture
- Animation
- Rapport, satisfaction and compliance

The study of body language was defined as kinesics by Dr Ray Birdwhistell (30). In his book he makes the following important observation: 'No body position or movement, in and of itself, has a precise meaning.' Therefore no single gesture or act can be interpreted in isolation. All signals, both verbal and non-verbal, must be interpreted together in order to establish context.

Having said this, in order to learn any language, we first learn the meaning of its individual constituents, then how to combine them to form more complex messages. In the same manner, it is reasonable to establish the meaning attributed to individual non-verbal signals in order to understand the meaning of complex patterns of communication.

In terms of managing PIA, such an understanding will allow strategies to be tailored in such a way that all aspects of communication are congruent and an overwhelming message of non-threat is delivered.

3.1 Proxemics

Edward Hall was the first to describe the phenomenon of proxemics in humans. Proxemics is the branch of knowledge that deals with the amount of space that people feel it necessary to set between themselves and others. A full original account can be found in Hall's book, *The Hidden Dimension*, first published in 1966 (31). In his text he defines four specific distances we adopt in everyday life. These are *Intimate*, *Personal*, *Social* and *Public*, each with a *close* and *far* phase. In addition, Hall makes a point in stating that the distance people establish and maintain with others is decisively influenced by a single factor – their feelings towards each other at the time.

Naturally, there will be slight variance in terms of these zones due to inter-individual idiosyncrasies and the fluidity in any interaction.

3.1.1 Intimate Distance

Close Phase: 0–6 Inches

Contact is possible with all parts of the body. In the absence of direct contact, the presence of another is easily apparent with all senses engaged and heightened due to proximity. Visualisation may be possible. If focus is achieved, any image formed will be greatly enlarged and distorted. Vocalisation as a communication is largely unnecessary as this distance is reserved for the most intimate interaction.

Far Phase: 6–18 Inches

Contact is easily possible with arms and hands. All sensations are engaged to a lesser degree but still active. Visualisation is possible but distorted. Whispering is the chosen form of verbal communication as it fits best with this proximity. This distance is only utilised with those who have a close intimate relationship. When forced into such proximity in public with strangers, a clear pattern of behaviour signalling that this proximity is not wanted will be deployed. This includes going rigid, turning our ventral aspect away from others and avoiding eye contact. Any public contact of this nature will usually stimulate a clear apology.

3.1.2 Personal Distance

Close Phase: 1.5–2.5 Feet

The implied sensation of someone being this close is dictated by what one can physically do to the other person. At this distance it is possible to contact and grip another person with arms and hands. Vision is normalised although straining of the eyes is still apparent. Those with an intimate relationship can be this close but in Western society, it would feel uncomfortable if they were a stranger.

Far Phase: 2.5–4 Feet

This equates to keeping someone at arm's length. This distance is anatomically defined as starting at the touching limit in terms of reach for one individual, and extends to the touching limit of two individuals reaching out towards each other. This is the limit or boundary for any potential physical domination in form of contact or an attack. Smell and temperature have become redundant. Vocalisation is of moderate volume. Vision is clear, detailed and accommodation effortless.

This is the standard proximity for conversation between two individuals. The distance may be closed slightly if there are others around and if further privacy with regards to verbal communication is required (32).

3.1.3 Social Distance

At either close or far phases, you are unable to touch the person you are communicating with and cannot physically dominate or threaten them. Volume of speech is normal.

Close Phase: 4–7 Feet

This is the distance for impersonal business, interaction with work colleagues and those we share space with but are not friends with. It is the distance for social interaction with unfamiliar individuals. Standing at this distance when another is seated generates a sense of being dominated in the seated individual.

Far Phase: 7–12 Feet

This is a more formal, less personal distance. It is the distance commonly encountered in the office setting between a superior seated behind their desk and the subordinate positioned in front of it. At this distance and its extreme, there is a necessity for greater eye contact in order to avoid appearing dismissive or disinterested. When eye contact is disengaged, it is a comfortable distance at which there is no compulsion to communicate. It offers some privacy if it is desired without appearing rude. Speech will need to be slightly louder than standard and can be overheard by others.

3.1.4 Public Distance

Close Phase: 12–25 Feet

This is the boundary for human flight distance, which is the point at which a potential for threat is sensed. In the animal kingdom, if another animal or human attains such proximity they will seek to avoid being attacked by moving away if at all possible. It is also the distance at which, if an animal cannot retreat, it will confront any perceived threat and aggressively defend itself. Vocalisation is louder than standard. Changes in vocalisation and syntax occur in order to compensate for any effect of distance on communication. This distance is generally used when lecturing or teaching.

Far Phase: 25 Feet or More

This is often deployed by people of status, and is the distance used for public figures of importance. Some animals will approach to this point then stop and move away. Cadence of speech must be reduced, volume of speech increased and other aspects of communication accentuated to compensate for a loss in clarity resulting from the distance involved.

In explanation for his chosen classification of proxemics, Hall wrote:

> Behind every classification system lies a theory or hypothesis about the nature of the data and their basic patterns of organization. The hypothesis behind the proxemic classification system is this: it is in the nature of animals, including man, to exhibit behavior which we call territoriality. In so doing, they use the senses to distinguish between one space or distance and another. The specific distance chosen depends on the transaction; the relationship of the interacting individuals, how they feel, and what they are doing. The four-part classification system used here is based on observations of both animals and men. Birds and apes exhibit intimate, personal, and social distances just as man does.

Hall also makes it clear that these distances are based upon Western society, and that other cultures differ significantly in their chosen distances and the meaning attributed to proximity.

In terms of utilising this information when interacting with an anxious child in order to optimally manage PIA, it is clear that clinicians should avoid crowding the child as this will be perceived as threatening. An understanding that a boundary exists and that the effects of seeking close proximity need to be monitored carefully is of great benefit to everyone working with children.

Rapport and a meaningful connection should be sought before moving from a public to social distance at around 12 feet or 4 metres. As stated above, a clinician moving through the boundary between these two will inevitably encounter the *flight distance* and trigger an increased sense of threat in a child, *unless rapport has been established or a more powerful counter signal of non-threat has been deployed in advance.* Once rapport is established, Hall's research shows that there is an inverse linear relationship between distance and an observer's perception of positive attitude illustrated by and towards the communicator (33). So, the closer you are, the more positively your behaviour and you as an individual will be perceived, as long as you are seen in a positive light and rapport has been established.

This is the phenomenon delineated by expectancy violations theory (EVT) described in detail in Section 5.5.1. This theory outlines the phenomenon whereby individuals predict expected patterns of behaviour in individuals they are observing or interacting with (34). These expectations will be based upon the myriad of rules regarding interpersonal behaviour. EVT seeks to study the positive and negative impact of any deviation from what has been predicted or is expected. The theory outlines the potential for such violations, in the presence of rapport and positive status or regard, defined in EVT as one's valence, to further enhance rapport and, under some circumstances, increase compliance. An understanding of EVT and proxemics offers an opportunity to disproportionately enhance rapport building by intentionally committing an *expectancy violation.* An example would be to deliberately breach the perimeter of what would normally be an acceptable or expected distance, such as entering the child's personal space.

A clinician's role may necessitate physical contact. This may grant an opportunity for a proxemic expectancy violation. An example might be holding the child's hand to check their name band or jokingly suggesting that you like their shoes, then positioning yourself side by side with your foot next to theirs while asking if their shoes might fit you. Such activities grant an excuse for entering personal and intimate space. In the presence of established rapport and positive valence, a violation of this nature will almost invariably further accelerate rapport building and enhance positive valence.

As a counter to this, an expectancy violation of this nature in the absence of rapport or where there is *negative* valence is likely to damage rapport building and increase anxiety.

In summary, we can see the importance of proxemics and EVT in the management of anxious children. Hall's work grants understanding, allowing us to predict negative responses to proximity, adjust our approach and avoid aggravating the anxiety response further. In parallel to this, EVT offers an incredibly powerful yet covert technique that enhances rapport building and the generation of positive valence, both of which significantly contribute as part of any anxiety management strategy.

3.2 Height

Height is well recognised as a means of asserting dominance in the animal kingdom. In the extreme, a dominant animal will stand over the submissive participant who will roll over and expose their ventral aspect, so exposing the areas of the body that would be targeted in a physical assault, such as the front of the neck. In doing this the dominant animal asserts their position within the hierarchy and the submissive animal signals their acceptance of this by making themselves more vulnerable to attack. An example of similar behaviour in humans is the symbolic act of kneeling or prostrating before a king or queen (35).

When working with anxious children, an understanding of this aspect of interaction is of vital importance. Children are predominantly shorter than adults. An anxious child who is confronted by an adult will inevitably feel an increased sense of vulnerability because of the difference in height. Under these circumstances the experienced clinician understands the value of crouching down to reach the same eye level as the child. In so doing, any negative influence of height is completely avoided. Taking this manoeuvre to its extreme, with an extremely anxious child, positioning yourself lower than the child by sitting on the floor can further reduce any sense of vulnerability or potential threat. This can be the difference between a child seeking to escape from the interaction or being comfortable enough to interact with the clinician, connect with them and start to build rapport.

3.3 Eye Contact

There is a socially accepted norm relating to eye contact. Having said this, what is accepted can vary significantly from one culture to the next.

In Western society, staring is not the standard approach. We stare at 'things' not at people, so staring at another individual implies the recipient is not a person and is not recognised as having the status that being a person brings. As such it belittles them and reduces their standing. Staring can act as a precursor to a rebuke or some other negative signal. It can also pose a question in and of itself, such as the glare a waiter receives if they remove a customer's half-full coffee cup before they have finished drinking. The glare says, 'What the hell are you doing'?

In general, however, eye contact will be limited to short glances of 3–10 seconds. These glances tend to be more frequent when listening as opposed to speaking, conforming to a ratio of about 3:1 respectively (36).

An individual who is speaking will often look away at the beginning of a sentence or utterance and look up when that part of their speech has finished. They then look away again when embarking on the next element of their interaction or continue looking up and holding eye contact, communicating that they have finished. Eye contact and frequency of glances is heavily influenced by proximity or proxemics. When there is significant distance between individuals who are communicating, eye contact is desired to reaffirm the connection, and as a consequence, glances will be significantly more intense. Prolonged eye contact in close proximity creates discomfort and can generate a sense of anxiety, so eye contact will become less frequent under these circumstances unless intimacy has been established. An extreme example of this is seen if two strangers are forced into close proximity. Under such circumstances they will *actively* avoid eye contact. Eye contact brings with it the imperative to recognise the other as a sign of social respect and acknowledgment of their existence. If eye contact is made under such circumstances, an individual will often fulfil this responsibility by producing a tepid smile, almost stating, 'Apologies for making eye contact. Now that I have, I must recognise your existence but I don't intend to bother you' (37, 38). This is all very interesting, but what is the relevance with regards to the management of PIA?

We can see that excessive eye contact can generate anxiety. Equally, reduced levels of eye contact will tend to communicate disinterest or that you are hiding something. If a child or family member feels that you are disinterested, it will significantly damage rapport. If they feel you are hiding something, both rapport and their trust in you may be damaged. When levels of eye contact are increased without becoming excessive, research shows that it will be appraised in a positive manner (39) and will increase compliance (40).

So, we should attempt to maintain our gaze at, or just above, normal levels in order to communicate attentiveness, enhance rapport and increase compliance. Excessive eye contact and staring should be avoided as it has the potential to communicate threat, dehumanise the recipient and increase anxiety levels.

An exception to this rule might be where a clinician is working with an autistic child who actively avoids visual contact as part of their normal behavioural routine. In such a situation it may be appropriate for the clinician to deviate from their own socially acceptable norm and adopt the same pattern of eye contact as the patient. This might feel odd, intuitively rude or dismissive for the clinician, yet it avoids causing discomfort or additional anxiety for the child.

Some children may feel shy or actively avoid eye contact with a view to pretending you are not there, or because they have attained the point of freeze–flight–fight. Under such circumstances eye contact is still required to avoid being dismissive or secretive, but it is wise to avoid prolonged or excessive contact. Intermittent glances will ensure optimum communication.

In summary, eye contact has considerable influence in the management of anxiety; therefore, understanding how it might be used to optimise communication is essential.

3.4 Facial Expression

Humans are exquisitely sensitive to the facial expressions of others. These expressions encompass a myriad of potential combinations and messages they may communicate. Considering that the face is arguably *the* most expressive aspect of our body, facial expressions have the potential to effect significant influence in the management of PIA.

The manner in which facial expression can be utilised in the management of PIA, despite the complexities of facial expression, is relatively simple. There are a number of universally recognised facial expressions. These are happiness, sadness, anger, fear, disgust and surprise (41, 42). When interacting with an anxious child, clinicians should utilise facial expressions that fit with a happy, calm and relaxed state, to further contribute to a non-threat message directed towards their patients. With this in mind, it is worth noting that it is relatively easy for our own personal experiences in the form of minor negative day-to-day irritations to result in facial expressions that reflect a sense of frustration or annoyance. Naturally, such expressions do not fit with efficiently communicating non-threat. Understanding this allows us to monitor our own experiences and adjust for any suboptimal influence they may have in the management of PIA.

3.5 Head Movement

In utilising our facial expressions to communicate, it is inevitable that positioning and movement of the head itself will contribute to the messages we send.

Birdwhistell described how the positions adopted by the head mark different points in the structure of conversation (43). These positions may be arbitrary and specific to the individual but are nevertheless consistent. Other positions are generic and culture-specific such as in Western American culture where individuals will often raise the head slightly, marking the end of their turn to communicate and signalling that they have finished speaking. These positions are interesting but it is only when they are indicative of attention or a lack of attention that they are important in the management of PIA. Positions or movements such as looking completely or slightly away or down with the head can be suggestive of disinterest and will have a negative impact on rapport building. Positions that communicate increased levels of attention and interest will naturally have the opposite effect.

Nodding the head during interaction has clearly been shown to significantly increase rapport and positively influence appraisal of the communicator by the observer (44). So, consistently facing an anxious child should signal interest and nodding appropriately will enhance rapport.

3.6 Posture

3.6.1 Tension and Relaxation

The degree of tension or relaxation we display has been shown to indicate our attitude towards others and is inevitably part of the message we send. In simple terms, it has been shown that we tend to either relax a lot or very little when interacting with those we dislike. Extreme tension usually indicates a threatening situation.

In evaluating this aspect of body language, we can see that a suitable intermediate level of muscle tone is most suited to optimal management of PIA. This is consistent with positive appraisal of the patient by the clinician and avoids any suggestion of hostility or anxiety (45).

3.6.2 Torso Angle

A study observing the influence of emotionally stimulating images showed that individuals will lean towards pleasant images and away from unpleasant images (46). Utilising the same mechanism of appraisal and in so doing sending an implied message, when appraising interactions between clinician and patient, leaning towards a patient has been shown to enhance rapport significantly, and leaning away has been shown to have a negative impact (44).

These findings may explain the negative impact that leaning away from a patient has with regards to rapport building. Alternative explanations for the positive influence of leaning towards a patient include imparting an increased sense of interest; displaying increased attentiveness; and generating a positive proxemic influence by reducing the effective distance between clinician and patient.

3.6.3 Open and Closed Posture

Crossing our arms or legs covers our ventral aspect and creates a barrier between the individual and everything else. This can be perceived as a defensive posture by those observing. Research shows that an open position positively influences rapport and a closed position is perceived negatively (44, 47). Additionally, crossed arms appear to have a greater negative influence on rapport than crossed legs. This may be due to their impact in terms prominence within our visual field during interaction.

3.6.4 Interactive Orientation

While defining Postural Indicators of Relationships, Albert Scheflin described two basic body orientations that a pair of individuals will adopt while communicating (48). These are the Vis-à-vis and the Parallel position. The position adopted is dictated by the relationship between the individuals and the task to be completed. Vis-à-vis is adopted during an exchange of information and commonly encountered in a teacher–student or in a doctor–patient exchange. Characteristically this arrangement requires both individuals to participate in communication for the position to remain functional. The Parallel position tends to be adopted when two individuals join each other in a task, the completion of which only requires the engagement of one of them. An example would be standing side-by-side in support of each other while engaging a third party in an argument or sitting side-by-side while one reads a story. For both of these positions there is a proxemic imperative in that effective verbal communication between two individuals in this orientation will require closing the distance between them. Of note, it is often the case that two individuals in the Vis-à-vis position who are communicating in public will move closer and more towards an angulated position if they wish to secure an increased level of privacy. This probably reflects the degree of comfort this position allows as opposed to the Vis-à-vis position when in close proximity. We should note the Vis-à-vis positioning associated with close proximity is a position adopted during confrontation and aggression. This may be the aetiology of discomfort often experienced in such an orientation and the reason the angulated position is adopted in a social setting.

Our preference for certain interactive orientations can be seen in research conducted by Robert Sommer (31, 49). Sommer studied the effect of seating position around a table on communication. The results are quite striking and show that communication is more frequent when individuals are positioned at the same corner of the table, at 90-degrees to each other, rather than opposite each other or side-by-side. Communication between individuals sitting together at the corners was twice as likely as that between individuals sat side-to-side. Side-by-side communication was in turn three times more common than communication when in a face-to-face position across the table. So, communication when at 90-degrees was *six times* more likely than when face-to-face. Again, these results are thought to reflect our preference for a position that optimises communication in terms of proximity, allows eye contact and avoids the sense of confrontation generated by a face-to-face interaction.

In terms of managing PIA, an understanding of these elements of non-verbal interaction allows us to utilise the Vis-à-vis position at a distance when imparting or extracting information and adopting an angulated interactive orientation in order to reduce the potential sense of threat when dealing with an anxious child. We can also see the benefit of adopting a parallel arrangement when attempting to generate a sense of teamwork or looking to work together to overcome a problem. The side-by-side or parallel position also offers an opportunity to enhance rapport building as a consequence of the proxemic expectancy violation this interactive position requires.

3.6.5 Mirroring

Mirroring was described by Albert Scheflin in terms of congruence and non-congruence of stance (48). From his research, Scheflin describes how adopting an identical or mirrored posture to the person or persons you are interacting with signals agreement or acceptance.

Although mirroring is a marker of congruence, evidence suggests that its impact on compliance and rapport is both subtle and inconsistent. As such, the efficacy of mirroring a child's posture and the physical practicalities of an adult attempting such a manoeuvre, are such that its value as a technique in the management of PIA is questionable. Attempts to mirror that are overt and easily detected may have a negative impact on communication.

3.6.6 Frame of Dominant Orientation

People orientate their body towards a frame of space that contains their main and long-term focus of interest. This frame of space is known as their *frame of dominant orientation* (50, 51).

The frame of dominant orientation is indicated by the ventral aspect of the body. There are three sections of the body in this respect and these are the legs and pelvis, the torso and then the head. As the legs and pelvis more dominantly set the limits of the positioning of the torso, and in turn the torso sets the limits of orientation of the head, the direction of the legs and pelvis have the greatest influence in dictating the frame of dominant orientation in comparison to the torso and head. The next most influential is the torso, then the head in turn. So, when a clinician's legs and pelvis are pointing towards a desk and computer, while their torso and head are rotated at 90-degrees to face the patient, the frame of dominant orientation is maintained towards the desk and computer. This indicates to the onlooker that, although they have acknowledged the patient's presence and engaged them, the clinician's main interest and intended long-term focus is the desk and computer. Equally, rotating the head towards an individual or activity while the torso and head remain in-line with another frame of space suggests only a passing interest. The frame of dominant orientation remains elsewhere. Alternatively, when a clinician moves their frame of dominant orientation away from an activity or object they have prioritised towards the patient, they signal that the patient is more important and has become the primary and long-term focus for the clinician. This increases the expressed attentiveness of the clinician which has been shown to be a factor in positively influencing rapport.

An understanding of this aspect of body language is of vital importance to the process of rapport building and the management PIA. It has been shown that the orientation of the body towards a subject during eye contact positively influences their attitude towards the observer (33). Additionally, in appreciating this subtlety in communication, a clinician can intentionally shift the perceived main focus of interest *away* from an anxious child with a view to granting them some space in order for them to calm down.

So, in managing PIA, we can appreciate there may be times when communicating intense interest and focus is desirable in order to enhance rapport, and other instances when choosing to intentionally signal a clear disinterest, will be preferable as it will reduce any sense of threat and allow an anxious child the space and time to calm down.

3.7 Animation

Tone and relaxation are important in the way you move and what this communicates. Clinicians should be moderately relaxed as they move. The signal this sends is that of an individual who is comfortable with the situation – *not* concerned or anxious. Anxiety is generally displayed by fidgeting and participation in redundant movements or idiosyncratic rituals such as pulling an ear lobe or scratching the nose (45). These are the physical equivalents of saying 'Um' and 'Er' and illustrate uncertainty or anxiety.

If one takes this to an optimal extreme, it is quite striking when there is a paucity of movement and complete absence of these ritualistic behaviours. The onlooker will often detect and be aware of this without it being at the forefront of conscious appraisal. Despite this 'void' in behaviour registering on what might be described as a subliminal level or in the pre-conscious, it will attract and hold their attention.

When married to the optimisation of all other aspects of interpersonal communication, appropriate forms of animation including the intentional deployment of such a 'void' can help to secure and maintain an external focus of attention, enhance rapport building and contribute to the generation of a positive and therapeutic clinician–patient relationship (52).

3.8 Relational Communication, Satisfaction and Compliance

There is an association between patient satisfaction and compliance (53). As a consequence, many have sought to understand satisfaction and its correlates with a view to informing practice and securing compliance more effectively. Burgoon defined the conglomerate of influences on satisfaction and compliance as relational communication. Her research suggests the most significant predictor of *patient satisfaction* is a clinician's perceived *receptivity*. Additional influences on patient satisfaction include *openness, interest, willingness to listen, involvement, warmth, similarity, equality* and displaying *some formality*.

In this context receptivity refers to the clinician's perceived level of interest in the patient themselves, what they are concerned about and what they are saying. Its presence implies acceptance and rapport. Similarity is seen where individuals reciprocate agreement, empathy, understanding, similar values and exchange personal information. They will mirror each other in terms of clothes, mannerisms and accents. It is worth highlighting the association with some formality. As this research study was conducted within an adult population, it should be noted that adults may expect a degree of formality in a clinical setting, while children may find formality intimidating. As such, avoiding formality may be better for the child with a view to optimising the management of PIA.

Compliance was only weakly linked to *similarity* and the *patient's affective satisfaction*, suggesting the relationship between them and any influence may be indirect. Affective satisfaction is characterised by patients feeling accepted, free to disclose information and that they are being taken seriously (54).

So, we can see clearly that body language can significantly and positively contribute to the successful management of PIA.

Key Points

- Personal space is broadly and stereotypically structured. An understanding of space and intentionally negotiating your position within such space is essential.
- Expectancy violations in the presence of positive valence and rapport will likely further enhance rapport and valence.
- Minimise any difference in height where possible.
- Look to establish and maintain moderate eye contact to communicate attentiveness and honesty. Readjust if eye contact appears to aggravate anxiety.
- Adopt a genuinely positive expression. Smile whenever possible and appropriate.
- Nod in response to patient communication.

- Adopt a positive lean towards those you are communicating with.
- Adopt an open posture with arms and legs uncrossed.
- Legs, torso and head should point towards the patient. Make the patient your frame of dominant orientation.
- Patterns of communication that grant a qualitative overview signalling receptivity, interest, willingness to listen, involvement, openness, warmth, similarity and equality may increase satisfaction and possibly compliance.

Verbal Communication

4

Verbal communication refers to all aspects of speech including linguistic and paralinguistic elements. Linguistic communication refers to the selection and integration of words into sentences and their literal or implied meaning. Paralinguistic communication encompasses all qualitative characteristics of speech. These qualitative elements often grant context and can exert a significant if not a dominant influence in dictating a recipient's interpretation and response. Qualitative elements include the tone, volume, tonal quality and cadence of speech. Aspects of verbal communication appraised in this section include:

- Paralinguistics
- Influence
- Therapy
- Conversational suggestion
- Utilisation and two-level communication theory
- Positive and negative vocabulary
- Positive pre-emptive interpretation
- Dynamic transition

4.1 Paralinguistics

Paralinguistics refers to the qualitative or vocal communication in speech that does not come from the words or verbal content. This includes volume, rate, tone, timbre, pauses, silences and other idiosyncrasies. For those unfamiliar with the term timbre, it refers to the quality of sound that is distinct from the other elements such as tone and volume.

Paralinguistics exert an exceptionally powerful if not dominant influence in communication. This is perfectly illustrated in Albert Mehrabian's statement, 'when vocal information contradicts verbal, vocal wins out' (45). To illustrate his point he sites sarcasm, defining it as 'a message in which the information transmitted vocally contradicts the information transmitted verbally.' The vocal content representing the intended message is invariably negative while the verbal content in isolation, would signal an equal and opposite positive message. An example would be to say, 'Yeh! He's really amazing.' When this is stated sarcastically, on the face of it the verbal message or words read in isolation would communicate a positive. However, the vocal elements that are overlaid when sarcasm is being deployed indicate the intended message is in fact the opposite. That he's not in the least bit amazing.

4.2 Influence

With regards to communication outside of any specialist environment, paralinguistics associated with dominance include loudness, high tempo, responding quickly, initiating conversation, interrupting, and speaking more. Speaking louder, high tempo and quicker uptake of speaking turns suggest confidence and authority. Other than interruptions, all of these vocal patterns tend to create favourable impressions (55).

An additional paralinguistic influence on the impression we make when we speak includes making mistakes, unnecessary repetitions, stuttering, missing parts of words, forming incomplete sentences and the inclusion of 'ums', 'ahs' and 'errs'. The appearance of these are more frequent when we are anxious or uncomfortable and as such, depending on the circumstances, they may be perceived by the listener as evidence of anxiety, nerves, uncertainty or a lack of confidence.

When it comes to doctor–patient interactions, vocal intonation has significant influence. Softer, warmer and non-angry vocal tones produce higher ratings of satisfaction (54).

Clinicians who adopt the correct tone, provide the required information by speaking relatively quickly and without hesitation, speak smoothly, use appropriate volume and speak clearly, are perceived as significantly more competent (56).

So, we can see that appearing to be competent and confident while connecting with the patient and displaying appropriate levels of empathy and receptivity will likely result in optimal satisfaction.

4.3 Therapy

Anxiety states in general and PIA, are associated with an altered state of consciousness that renders an individual more receptive to suggestion and influence. As such, anxiety generates a unique opportunity to utilise therapy-based communication techniques with a view to managing and reducing anxiety. The paralinguistics commonly utilised during hypnotherapy are ideally suited to such situations as they can be deployed by covertly braiding highly influential behaviour modification techniques into normal conversation.

Such paralinguistic patterns are characterised by speech that is slow and clear, having a lowered calming tone and the adoption of a downward inflection at the end of each sentence, preferably timed to coincide with the recipient or patient breathing out. This pattern of communication reinforces the altered state and encourages adjustment of physiological parameters towards enhanced parasympathetic tone more commonly associated with calm and relaxation. In turn, this leads to a reduction in *sympathetic* tone more commonly associated with anxiety. Such a readjustment of physiology leads to a readjustment in psychological parameters and significantly contributes to the management and reduction of anxiety (57, 58).

4.4 Conscious, Preconscious/Subconscious and Unconscious Awareness

Freud described the existence of the conscious mind (Cs), preconscious mind (Pcs) and unconscious mind (Ucs). He defined the Cs as containing everything that we are aware of; the Pcs as everything that we are not currently aware of yet but can become conscious of if we so wished; and the Ucs containing information that is either inaccessible to the Cs or Pcs or only accessible with extreme difficulty (59). This organisation of consciousness and the mind continues to form a basis for discussion to this day. Many deploy the terms defined by Freud indiscriminately, and the term subconscious is often used interchangeably with the less familiar term, Pcs. With this in mind, to clarify, in the subsequent text Cs and Ucs are deployed as defined by Freud and the more familiar term subconscious (Scs) will be used to represent the less familiar Pcs.

The argument with regards to the nature of consciousness is ongoing, yet it is broadly suggested that processing within the conscious mind forms the *minority* of activity on a day to day basis. The majority of processing and initiation of any response takes place outside conscious awareness and attention. Although it is possible for us to become aware of some of this information by choosing to focus on it, there is far too much data for us to process *all* of it while still remaining functional. It would overload our conscious capacity. This is the concept of knowing something, yet not knowing that you know it until prompted to retrieve the information from the Pcs.

The processing of information outside conscious appraisal and the therapeutic opportunity this presents us with was highlighted in the publication by Rossi and Erickson in their description of Two-Level Communication Theory and the Microdynamics of Suggestion (60).

4.5 Two-Level Communication Theory

Over a prolonged period, Ernest Rossi worked with Milton Erickson and sought to both learn from him and analyse the techniques he deployed in his practice. Two-level communication was one of the techniques he documented. Rossi describes how the sentences we create are made up of words and phrases that if appraised in isolation will each have their own independent meaning and context. Under normal circumstances, the goal of conscious critical appraisal in communication is to discard the individual and literal associations of component words and phrases in favour of seeking the general context in each interaction. However, in the presence of an altered state of consciousness or trance, where dissociation and literalness are heightened, the literal meaning of individual words and phrases *may* be analysed in isolation by the Scs and Ucs and as a consequence they *can* play a significant role in facilitating responsive behaviour. Rossi defines this as Two-Level Communication Theory and describes how Erickson would deploy mundane dialogue, the only purpose of which was to fixate attention, while simultaneously braiding carefully selected therapeutic words and phrases within each sentence, so they might be covertly delivered to the Scs and Ucs for processing.

One of the best examples of two-level communication is the use of embedded suggestions, also referred to as the interspersal technique. Suggestions are placed within sentences and highlighted by deploying subtle vocal adjustments, such as a slight pause before their delivery or a change in cadence, volume or tone while delivering them. The subtlety in highlighting this content is enough to evade conscious critical appraisal, while ensuring they are noted, processed and acted upon by the Scs and Ucs.

So, if we accept that our mind processes much of the information we receive outside of conscious awareness, there are techniques we can utilise to intentionally and effectively evade conscious critical appraisal while delivering information directly to the Scs and Ucs for processing. If we accept that altered states of consciousness and trance are characterised by increased dissociation and literalness which facilitates responsive behaviour, then we are presented with a mechanism, techniques and conditions that favour the management of anxiety in general and more specifically PIA, which is characterised by increased vigilance and an increased propensity towards resistance.

4.6 The Microdynamics of Suggestion

In considering the phenomenon of trance, Rossi observed there were five stages of hypnotic trance induction and suggestion which he defined as follows.

Fixation of attention

This refers to attracting and maximally pre-occupying the recipient's attention.

De-potentiating conscious sets

This is the disruption of automated and stereotyped processes that are taking place within the conscious mind which include the capacity for conscious critical appraisal. Such processes are based upon past experience, learnt behaviour, preconceptions and assumed context. They can impede the narrowing of focus and represent an obstacle to the adoption of alternative, new perspectives and re-evaluation of a situation. In terms of anxiety management, a technique that might de-potentiate conscious sets might be an interaction that commands the maximum bandwidth of conscious appraisal. This may include an unexpected behaviour, the use of confusion, or presentation of an overwhelming volume of information, all of which are discussed in greater detail in later sections. Any such approach will disrupt conscious processes including the internal focus, negative rumination and dialogue associated with hypervigilance generated in response to perceived or potential threat. They will additionally contribute to fixating and narrowing attention and focus.

When conscious sets are de-potentiated, the frame of reference conscious sets provide is suspended. As a direct consequence an individual's understanding of what is happening, of their reality, is undermined. This generates a need to make sense of the situation which can only be met by the unconscious mind, as conscious processes are already maximally engaged.

Unconscious search

This is the process of seeking new associations within the unconscious mind with a view to making sense of the situation.

Unconscious process

Once associations and points of reference are identified, unconscious processing generates meaning and context.

Hypnotic response

After completing an unconscious search and processing, an autonomous response is formulated which is then delivered to the conscious mind. Once delivered to the conscious mind, there is the potential for this autonomous response to influence thinking, perspective and behaviour.

In understanding this framework for trance induction and the deployment of suggestion, we should note that trance phenomena are not exclusive to hypnotherapy. Quite the opposite, altered states of consciousness and trance phenomena including the enhanced dissociation and literalness they are associated with are natural phenomena that each and every one of us experiences every day. The practice of hypnotherapy simply utilises this phenomenon with a view to minimising resistance and maximising an individual's response to therapeutic intervention.

We should also note that this process of trance induction and suggestion is almost identical to that which is encountered in the management of PIA. When confronted with an anxious child undergoing medical intervention, we seek to reach them, fixate and command their full attention, de-potentiate the conscious processes associated with anxiety and hypervigilance, communicate non-threat and calm on multiple levels both verbally and non-verbally, attempt to stimulate an unconscious re-evaluation of the situation through suggestion and offer coping strategies, with a view to supporting a change in thinking, perspective and behaviour. When one understands that altered states of consciousness occur naturally, in the absence of formal trance induction, that anxiety states are associated with an altered state of consciousness and that children are more suggestable than adults, it is easy to appreciate the value of suggestion in the management of PIA. Additionally, when one considers the hypervigilance and resistance characteristic of the anxiety state, we can understand the value of braiding suggestions into regular conversation in order to generate a child-centred, dynamic, versatile and covert therapeutic intervention.

4.7 Conversational Suggestion

Under normal circumstances, a suggestion made in conversation is likely to have minimal influence unless the individuals involved have an established positive relationship, the influencer has significantly positive valence (discussed in the enhanced communication section) or the influencer has had training in one of the speaking therapies and is skilled in the art of suggestion. This latter skillset is of considerable interest and value in the management of PIA and anxiety states for the reason outlined above.

Stereotyped paralinguistic patterns of therapeutic communication can be utilised to draw attention at a subconscious level to therapeutic metaphor and suggestion, dispersed throughout normal conversation, which in turn has the potential to generate considerable influence. When this approach is deployed by a clinician who has positive valence and has taken time to established rapport, in the management of an anxious child who by definition is likely to be in an altered state and therefor hyper-suggestable, they can wield profound influence.

Suggestions can be incredibly simple, direct and literal such as; 'I expect you'll feel really hungry after this is done.' This might be helpful in a situation where nausea is a possibility. Suggesting the observer will be hungry has the potential to counter any nausea, as nausea and hunger as states are mutually exclusive and cannot coexist. Suggestions may be made to encourage any type of feeling, sensation or even a lack of sensation, with the outcome directly influenced by the quality of relationship between clinician and recipient.

In accepting the powerful influence conversational suggestion can exert we can appreciate there is also the potential to inadvertently deliver *negative* suggestions with unwelcome consequences. No medical professional would do this deliberately but in the absence of formal training in this area of communication skills, it can easily happen. A real-life example of this was the unforeseen consequence of an anaesthetist who told a particularly suggestible child they might feel dizzy and taste garlic as they administered an intravenous anaesthetic. Subsequently, this child became terrified of feeling dizzy and tasting garlic and refused all attempts to deliver intravenous anaesthesia. With this in mind, it is wise to carefully consider all that you say. If in doubt – leave it out.

4.7.1 Nature and Complexity of Suggestion

When it comes to suggestion delivered to an individual in an altered state, the majority of understanding we have stems from work in the field of hypnotherapy. Basic classification of suggestions defines simple, direct and literal suggestions such as the example above as *direct suggestions* as they are direct and overt by nature. They simply and directly suggest something will or will not happen. There is little subtlety and no attempt is made to evade conscious appraisal of the suggestion or avoid precipitating resistance as the direct consequence of the recipient resenting the fact they are being told what to do.

When managing an anxious child, resistance is likely if the recipient feels they are being dictated to, particularly if direct suggestions are deployed in an attempt to gain compliance with respect to an anxiogenic task or situation. Under these circumstances the deployment of a less direct, subtle or even covert approach is likely to be more successful. An example would be to utilise what are defined as *indirect suggestions*. Indirect suggestions are designed to achieve the same or similar response or outcome to direct suggestions, while avoiding simply telling the recipient what to do. There are different levels of complexity with regards to indirect suggestion, yet most are designed to generate the illusion of choice for the recipient in addition to delivering the suggestion itself and in so doing, they maximise the likelihood of compliance by minimising resistance. Naturally, as stated above, the response to any suggestion will depend on the recipient's positive appraisal of the clinician, the situation or their general disposition towards the suggested outcome. For example, a suggestion is unlikely to be successful in isolation if the clinician is not trusted, if the suggestion seeks to directly negate a survival-based response in the recipient, or if the suggestion would be completely unacceptable under any circumstances. It is important to grasp this baseline architecture of any situation where influence is sought through suggestion. Success requires rapport, a careful and often indirect stimulus towards the desired outcome, and most importantly an understanding of the boundaries within which the recipient functions.

Our understanding of indirect suggestion and their use stems predominantly from the extensive work of Milton Erickson, one of the most prominent hypnotherapists of the twentieth century. As a result, they are often referred to as Ericksonian suggestions and language patterns (61–64).

Indirect suggestions and Ericksonian language patterns that may be of particular use in the conversational management of anxious children and PIA include the following.

4.7.2 Permissiveness

Any direct suggestion can be made less dictatorial and more permissive by incorporating words such as 'might', 'may', 'possibly', 'perhaps', 'could', 'can'. This grants the recipient the sense that it is their choice whether they comply and that they maintain control over their decisions. Examples of this include; 'You might *find yourself feeling deeper and deeper relaxed.*' or 'When you feel the time is right for you, you might *start to feel really comfortable, more comfortable than you have felt before.*' and '*That pain in your arm is going to gradually fade away.* But only when you are ready.'

In all of these examples, the permissive element is written in standard text and the direct suggestion highlighted in italic. When spoken, the permissive element of the sentence should delivered as an obvious statement, understated and almost a 'throw away comment'. The direct suggestion should be delivered in a contrasting manner that is detectable at a subconscious level yet subtle enough to evade conscious appraisal. An example approach to managing this contrast would be to pause for a split second before the direct suggestion, then continue speaking in a minimally louder, slower and more eloquent manner. Naturally, if the contrast is too obvious it will attract attention, almost certainly arouse suspicion and stimulate conscious critical appraisal.

4.7.3 Imagination

Another way to generate an indirect suggestion is by *asking* the recipient if they can *imagine* what it feels like to be or to feel whatever you are suggesting, such as … calmer, more comfortable, more relaxed … than they have ever been before. As ever, the potency of these suggestions is dependent upon rapport, the recipient's altered state and the use of therapeutic language patterns.

4.7.4 Metaphor and Storytelling

This form of indirect suggestion utilises a story or metaphor as a proxy to represent and deliver the intended suggestion. Telling a story about someone feeling really calm, how this affects all of their senses and their breathing, represents an indirect suggestion when the listener identifies and connects with the story and the experience described within it. Describing a bright sunny day in a field of flowers with blossom floating on a gently cooling breeze can act as a metaphor for how you would like the recipient to feel. These suggestions should be as rich and elaborate as possible in order to fully engage the listener. Lastly, you would be correct in perceiving this approach as a simple form of guided imagery. It is worth noting that many behaviour and anxiety management techniques border on and overlap with others, reflecting the fluid and dynamic nature of all successful individualised management strategies.

4.7.5 Content Free Suggestions

Content free suggestions generate a potent highly person specific suggestion by drawing directly on the recipient's own resources without needing to know exactly what these are. This type of suggestion originates from the practice of Milton Erickson who commented that there was no real need to dig around and dissect a patient's past life in order to find a solution for their current problems, and that this was incredibly intrusive. An alternative was to make a broad content free suggestion related to the problem and allow the recipient to generate a personalised solution without the need for intrusion.

To illustrate this, consider the following examples utilising imagination to generate calm and relaxation. First, a clinician may ask the recipient to imagine they are on a beach, it is sunny with a cooling gentle breeze, they have sand between their toes, and they can hear the soft sounds of water lapping on the shoreline and children playing in the distance. This suggestion clearly specifies the parameters of the content and the resource in the form of positive memories the clinician is attempting to utilise. As such, it is restricted, has clear content and the clinician assumes that such a description represents a generic resource common to most individuals, including the recipient. I expect most of us would find this imagery relaxing; however there is always a possibility that the recipient may have strong negative associations with this imagery. Additionally, the recipient may possess a more powerful and heavily conditioned resource that would be far more effective in generating the desired emotional and cognitive state. Such a resource might be easy to establish by interviewing the recipient, but a simpler far more efficient means to ensure you connect with the most effective resources is to deploy a content free suggestion. An example might be to suggest the recipient imagines the most relaxing experience they have ever had, to remember how they felt, all of the sensations they experienced and the deep sense of calm and peace they experienced as a result. This second suggestion has minimal content and allows the recipient to connect with whatever resource suits them best. As such, this suggestion is also permissive. Naturally, this does not cater for someone who has no resources to draw upon. Appropriate management in the absence of resources will depend on the focused attention of the clinician, closely observing the recipient's responses as an index of success or failure. If any single approach is not working, a transition towards a more content-rich directive based on common stereotypical resources may be more appropriate. It may be that a completely different approach is required. This real-time, dynamic and critical appraisal of the recipient's response is key to any behaviour management strategy, particularly the management of PIA.

4.7.6 Embedded Suggestion/Interspersal of Suggestions

Embedding or interspersing suggestions throughout normal mundane conversation is a means to deploy the phenomenon described in the section on two-level communication theory. As stated, highlighting these suggestions by deploying subtle vocal adjustments, such as a slight pause before their delivery or a change in cadence, volume or tone while delivering them ensures they are noted, processed and acted upon by the Scs and Ucs, while evading conscious critical appraisal. Such techniques maximise the delivery and potential for therapeutic intervention while minimising the chances of resistance.

4.7.7 Implication

Implication is where a statement is made, the listener processes the statement and *infers* something *by association*. As such, it is a form of indirect suggestion.

The Cambridge Dictionary defines implication in this context as 'an occasion when you seem to suggest something without saying it directly' (65). Of particular relevance is the Merriam-Webster dictionary definition outlining the relationship between the two propositions in implication. This relationship dictates that when one proposal or suggestion is accepted, a second dependent proposition is inferred and also be accepted (66).

The value of implication in suggestion and behaviour management is the ability to imply something without saying it. If what is stated, once it is consciously and critically appraised, is held to be true and as such is accepted, what is inferred will tend to be accepted without conscious critical appraisal. In clinical practice, our ability to utilise implication is critically dependent on our ability to select a stated proposition that is reliably accepted and will in turn reliably generate the second inferred proposition we wish to deliver. We should recognise that acceptance of any stated proposition and the potency of implication is significantly influenced by rapport and the clinician's ability to predict the recipient's response.

The efficacy of implication can be illustrated by its use in the management of PIA generated by past traumatic medical interventions. The primary step in managing PIA in this situation might be to validate the negative experiences by openly acknowledging them. If the clinician then states that, as a direct consequence of appreciating past difficulties, they intend to approach and do things differently, this implies, and the observer may infer, that the consequent experience will *also* be different. It might even be a positive one. The goal in deploying this technique is to generate motivation, enhance compliance and undermine resistance. Naturally, failure to deliver an improved outcome, may undermine rapport, trust and reinforce negative patterns of behaviour.

An example of this approach would be for a child with PIA associated with the experience of intravenous drugs that are injected quickly, such as anaesthetic induction agents. If the clinician states they know and understand what they don't like, why they don't like it and that as a consequence they plan to give the drug slowly, this recognition and validation of the child's past experiences is likely to enhance rapport, and implies by doing it differently the experience may also be different. It is worth noting there is an opportunity for a clinician to further enhance the potency of this strategy by braiding in additional behaviour modification techniques such as asking the child to watch and make sure that only a small amount of drug is injected at a time. This will command the child's full and external focus of attention, which in turn disrupts negative internal dialogue, engages participation in the very process that generated anxiety before, and offers the child a sense of control or mastery.

In summary, implication is a form of indirect suggestion. As such, when deployed as part of an anxiety management strategy, it represents a highly effective tool for minimising resistance and maximising compliance. We should note that implication is not exclusively a verbal technique as anything that is observed or experienced can imply *something*. We should always expect whatever the observer infers to be significantly influenced by their current experiential, emotional and cognitive state. For a child who suffers from PIA, their state will tend to be dominated by fear, self-preservation, suspicion and resistance. With this in mind, when managing such children, we should seek to ensure all communication is congruent, is consistent with and therefore implies an absence of threat, that every*thing* and every*one* in the immediate proximity are calm. If we achieve this, we will generate an environment that challenges stereotypical patterns of thought, feelings and behaviour generated in response to PIA, and nurture those that are consistent with calm, security, trust and compliance. As outlined in previous sections, we know that much of the processing that underpins evaluation and response in such situations takes place outside consciousness and that carefully selected patterns of communication can evade critical appraisal and generate considerable therapeutic influence. By understanding communication techniques and the manner in which communication is processed, a clinician will be empowered to utilise all opportunities for communication en masse, with a view to intentionally sending one single, congruent and overwhelmingly positive therapeutic message. When this is achieved, the influence on a recipient's response and behaviour will be profound.

4.7.8 Utilisation

Milton Erickson proposed an approach to therapy that differed significantly from the use of ritualistic and formal interactions. His approach was to adopt a natural, conversational style and most importantly accepted the realities and responses of his patients. This approach allowed the patient's responses to dictate the approach itself in real-time, in a fluid, responsive and dynamic way. As such, every interaction was bespoke, tailored to the individual's needs. This became known as *utilisation theory* where all responses, even resistance to therapeutic intervention, are seen as positive, as potential energy that can be utilised and re-directed in order to achieve a therapeutic and positive outcome. Naturally the success of such a strategy is dependent on the ability of the clinician to embrace whatever response is made and integrate this into their approach in real-time, conversationally and naturally as the interaction evolves (67, 68).

The power of utilisation lies in accepting the patient's reality and responses as being 'OK' rather than the clinician treating them as an obstacle to achieving any preconceived outcome. In so doing, the clinician implies they understand and accept the patient's reality, feelings and wishes and see them as part of the solution. The patient is not 'wrong', they are 'right'. This simple yet fundamental step redefines the relationship between clinician and patient as one where they are working together rather than against each other. As such the patient is a part of the solution, a member of the team, rather than the passive recipient of therapeutic intervention. Additionally, as a direct consequence, a sense of equity in the therapeutic process is generated, rapport is enhanced, resistance minimised and compliance is nurtured.

To illustrate the use of utilisation, we can highlight the part it plays in the example used to illustrate implication. For the child who experiences anxiety and displays resistance towards the administration of intravenous medication, rather than seeing their response as an inconvenience and something to be overpowered, the clinician has the opportunity to accept the behaviour and utilise it as part of an anxiety management strategy. In our chosen example, such utilisation can be seen when the clinician engages and redeploys the child's energies in watching the process of drug administration very carefully and making sure that the medication is injected in the correct way. In accepting the child's reality and behaviour in this manner and utilising their response as part of the management strategy, the clinician commands their full and external focus of attention, disrupts negative internal dialogue, engages participation in the very process that generated anxiety, and offers the child a sense of control or mastery.

In summary, utilisation is simple, yet immensely powerful. It is not just a management strategy, it is a generic disposition. In understanding its use and value, we can see how and why it should be a core competency, braided into standard practice (69).

4.7.9 Use of Negatives

One form of utilisation is the deployment of a negative with a view to generating the opposite response. An example might be, 'Don't relax until you are completely ready.' This approach seeks to accept, encourage and utilise resistance with a view to turning it upon itself. Under such circumstances, suggesting the opposite response to the one we are truly seeking, should result in the response we are looking for. It is worth noting that by accepting resistance, the patient's sense of autonomy is supported, even if in truth it is an illusion of choice.

4.8 Positive and Negative Vocabulary

With an understanding of suggestion, comes an appreciation that some words are inextricably associated with an emotional, cognitive and behavioural response. An example is the word 'pain'.

In the presence of anxiety, a child is likely to perceive the environment as hostile until proven otherwise and display a heightened sensitivity towards all communication, particularly negative words or comments. An example of a phrase with negative potential might be, 'Kiss your child goodbye.' If this phrase is used as a parent leaves the room after anaesthetic induction prior to surgery, there is the potential for the parent to infer they will never see their child again. Another example might be an anaesthetist telling a child that they are going to be 'put to sleep'. As this phrase is commonly used by veterinary practitioners to describe terminating the life of a sick animal, its use may understandably generate significant anxiety. In essence then, any communication that *can* be perceived as indicating something negative, almost certainly will and as such, it is best to avoid using any word or phrase that has the slightest chance of being perceived as anything less than overwhelmingly and indisputably positive.

All clinicians have a situation-based vocabulary they use on a regular basis. As such, it should be relatively simple to evaluate the anxiogenic potential of all of the words and phrases we commonly deploy, from the patient's perspective. If it is possible for any of them to be perceived as negative, then it is worth replacing them with an unequivocally positive alternative. When doing this, there may not be a clear, diametrically opposed substitute. An example of such a situation might be when using the word 'nausea'. There is no diametrically opposed positive alternative to nausea that will avoid the suggestion of feeling sick. Attempting to communicate its opposite by stating; 'you will not feel nauseated', often fails as the listener tends to ignore the beginning of the sentence, while focusing on and processing the word 'nauseated'. For words of this nature, the solution is to avoid them altogether by using an alternative that indicates a positive state that is incompatible with the one we are trying to avoid. Taking the example of nausea, this might be to suggest the listener will feel hungry, as the state of being nauseated is incompatible with that of feeling hungry. In this way, we abandon a negative conversational suggestion in favour of one that is positive.

With regards to words that are commonly utilised in practice, one such word that appears to be impossible to replace with a more positive alternative is the word 'needle'. It may be worth avoiding its use altogether unless the sharing of a comprehensive account of proceedings has positive cognitive therapeutic value. When seeking an alternative to the word pain, perhaps comments such as, 'I will give some medication that *should* ensure you are *comfortable*.' Naturally, making an outright promise to deliver a specified outcome is unwise. Failure to deliver on such a promise would undermine trust and rapport. With this in mind it is best to incorporate a degree of uncertainty within any discussion regarding expectations. This can be achieved by integrating words such as 'try' and 'should' when discussion any potential outcome.

4.9 Positive Pre-emptive Interpretation

Children are exquisitely sensitive to change. Exposure to unfamiliar or unpredictable situations can undermine their sense of security, generate anxiety and fear. Once fear and anxiety have been established, a child's response to sudden or marked changes in their surroundings or what they are experiencing will tend to be disproportionate and negative by default.

With this in mind, one aspect of managing PIA is *positive pre-emptive interpretation*. Most clinicians are familiar with aspects of practice that children commonly find disturbing, distressing or due to the sudden nature of the change they bring, can be startling. Prior to such an event, in advance of any potential negative evaluation, there is an opportunity for the clinician to pre-emptively label the experience in a positive way. This positive pre-emptive interpretation supports anxiety management in a number of ways. By warning the child that something is about to happen it makes their environment more predictable and less frightening. It offers a positive evaluation of the situation before any negative appraisal can be made, which undermines negative ideation and behaviour. Lastly, it suggests the clinician is familiar with what is happening, which enhances their credibility and nurtures trust.

As discussed in the section on positive and negative vocabulary, our options in selecting a positive pre-emptive alternate interpretation may not include a diametrically opposed term or phrase. One advantage when dealing with adjectives, is the option to choose an *abstract alternative* to describe a situation or experience. This grants an opportunity to engage the child's imagination and deploy humour. The more ridiculous or abstract the chosen alternative, the more engaging the process of establishing the connection between the situation and the adjective will be. In fact, using adjectives that are completely out of context is almost guaranteed to deliver the greatest amusement.

Again, using the example of the child receiving intravenous medication, we might suggest in advance that when the drug is injected, it might feel really '*pink*'.

By utilising one simple word in this manner, an *abstract alternative*, we *command* an *external focus* of attention, *disrupt* internal processes by deviating from expected behaviour, generate *confusion* which in turn stimulates an *internal search for clarity* and offer humour as a *coping strategy*. It is incredible that all of this can be achieved with a single word and at the same time as deploying a *positive pre-emptive interpretation*.

Another example might be when a child is being cannulated after local anaesthetic cream has been applied. Any experienced clinician will appreciate local anaesthetic cream can anaesthetise small nerves that transmit pain sensation while leaving larger nerves that transmit mechanical sensations unaffected. As such we know a patient will not sense any pain when a needle is introduced into the skin, yet they might still feel pressure or pushing on the skin and underlying structures. An anxious child will automatically fear that anything they feel will be pain, which may lead them to incorrectly label the sensations they experience. It is therefore wise to warn a child of the phenomena where pain is absent in isolation and provide an accurate and *positive pre-emptive interpretation* of what they will feel, which will be 'pressure or pushing'. If we take the time to explain this phenomenon, most children although sceptical find details of how the cream affects different nerves fascinating. To a child the phenomenon appears almost magical which is almost guaranteed to appeal.

As a last example, we can consider induction of anaesthesia with volatile anaesthetic. Volatile anaesthetics have a distinctive smell that to some are pleasant and others not quite so appealing. At the beginning of induction, the child is often breathing oxygen and nitrous oxide, there is little smell but a child will begin to feel lightheaded and may experience the sensation of 'pins-and-needles' in the skin. By telling the child that they are breathing what many refer to as 'laughing gas', by preceding these two words with a subtle pause and deliver them while utilising a therapeutic pattern of speech, we draw attention to the words and deliver a *positive indirect conversational suggestion*, an *implication* that they will laugh. If we wish, we can deploy humour by asking them what they think laughing gas will do. In the appropriate age group, we could also *positively pre-empt* their *interpretation* of the sensation of pins and needles at anaesthetic induction by stating that they may feel as if they are being tickled all over by pixies. Lastly, when the volatile anaesthetic is about to be administered, we can *pre-empt the change* in aroma and *positively interpret* it by warning them and suggesting it will 'just smell different'. This can be followed by a comment that it's a smell that you, the person delivering the anaesthetic, quite like. If you have established rapport with the child then this statement will represent a *positive conversational suggestion*.

4.10 Dynamic Transition

When one understands the method and power of conversational suggestion, it is worth highlighting one aspect of its delivery. The shift from regular 'normal' speech towards an intentionally therapeutic pattern of communication can exert therapeutic influence.

If a clinician moves smoothly and subtly from standard conversation to an 'altered' pattern, this change will tend to evade conscious evaluation by the recipient. In terms of Freud's delineation of consciousness, a subtle transition may evade conscious thought yet be noted and evaluated by the pre-conscious. As we have come to understand, this has the advantage of offering powerful influence while evading conscious critical evaluation and minimising the potential for resistance. If, alternatively, the clinician chooses to accentuate the transition from standard to therapeutic patterns by moving abruptly from one to the other, this will be detected, command the recipient's full attention and generate an intense external focus.

The choice to deploy an overt or covert approach will depend on the child and the circumstances. A covert approach may better suit situations where we wish to avoid inflaming the situation further, such as those where anxiety levels are already high, resistance is of particular concern and the recipient's coping strategies are limited. The overt approach may better suit situations where the recipient is cooperative and inquisitive, yet needs assistance in managing anxiety by diversion from an internal focus with negative ideation, towards an external focus and the management strategy on offer. An overt approach may also offer a means to command attention and assume control of any situation where multiple well-meaning individuals are unsuccessfully attempting to manage a child's anxiety.

Key Points

- Both vocal and verbal content significantly influence therapeutic outcome.
- When seeking to manage an anxious child or PIA, a clinician should speak with a warm, soft tone, normal or minimally raised volume and intermediate and assertively brisk cadence. They should speak confidently, avoiding idiosyncrasies that might indicate uncertainty and display immediacy by attentively responding to the patient.
- The ability to utilise a therapeutic voice, dynamic transition and conversational suggestion grants the capacity to wield considerable therapeutic influence as part of any anxiety management strategy.
- Clinicians should recognise the existence of altered states of consciousness, that patients are often in an altered state when anxious, and that this state enhances the potency of communication with and processing by the unconscious mind.
- In the presence of resistance, compliance is more likely achieved by deploying indirect or content free suggestions rather than more direct techniques.
- Suggestions can be both positive *and* negative.
- Clinicians should choose their words carefully and review the terms they commonly deploy, replacing those that may be perceived in a negative light with those that will likely generate a more predictably positive response.
- In any situation where sudden or marked changes are likely, the clinician should seek to pre-emptively interpret them in a positive light. This may require careful selection of an abstract alternative.
- It is clear that all of a child's responses, including resistance, are of great value and can be utilised in the process of communication and the provision of therapeutic support.

Enhanced Communication Strategies

As has been defined in previous sections, the ability to manage PIA is dependent on coping strategies, the ability to deploy them and whether the situation is such that they are adequate or are overwhelmed.

In addition, one must recognise that the fundamental characteristic of the anxiety state is an intense internal focus towards the negative feelings and thoughts precipitated by anxiety and the situation. The state then 'feeds' upon itself, reinforcing the emotions, feelings and thoughts that grow exponentially unless a successful management strategy is implemented or the pressure in terms of the anxiogenic stimulus is released.

Enhanced communication strategies offer solutions on one of three axes. These may be deployed in isolation or, as is often the case, in combination – acting in synergy to achieve the desired outcome. Strategies either disrupt internal focus, enhance rapport, or they offer a ready-made coping strategy.

In order to quickly delineate which of the techniques falls into which category the following key will be used:

IF – Intervention that disrupts Internal Focus

RB – Intervention that enhances Rapport Building

CS – Intervention that delivers a Coping Strategy

5.1 Internal Focus

In any interaction with an anxious child, a clinician must first reach and connect with them. To do this the characteristic internal focus must be disrupted. This will move the child's attention away from the negative appraisal of their situation, with negative thoughts and feelings causing negative patterns of behaviour and force a connection with the outside world. Generally speaking, the techniques that achieve this will often simultaneously command a re-appraisal of the outside world, and therefore the situation the child finds themselves in. An example would be incongruent behaviour that is extreme enough to command attention.

5.2 Rapport Building

This aspect of interaction may or may not come next, but certainly after a connection has been established. Rapport was defined in the earlier sections. There are many techniques to enhance rapport and additionally techniques that specifically enhance the quality or magnitude of rapport that is established. An example of this below is valence optimisation which seeks to enrich positive evaluation of the clinician with a view to further enhancing their potential influence in managing anxiety.

5.3 Coping Strategies

Coping strategies are utilised when one of three conditions exist. These include: when a child has no strategies of their own; if the strategies they have cannot sufficiently manage the situation at hand; or lastly, for whatever and often unknown reasons, they simply cannot deploy the strategies they have.

The ability to tell which of these is the problem in not important. Offering a coping strategy, often guided by an understanding of the child, and an appreciation of any positive resources they might have, should help to manage and may even reduce their anxiety. Experienced clinicians learn to rapidly deploy multiple strategies simultaneously and allow them to run in parallel. They will then observe and allow organic evolution of those achieving the desired therapeutic effect, while abandoning those that are not. This might appear an intimidating undertaking to those who are yet to explore anxiety management strategies. Be reassured, even those with the greatest expertise, will have started by deploying just one technique that happened to appeal to them in isolation, then adding to their repertoire over time.

It is worth making a clear point, that to deliver these techniques effectively and to appreciate which techniques are having the desired effect, the clinician, like the child, must be exclusively externally focused. There is little point attempting to connect with a child and deploy coping strategies if it is done at random with no reference to the child's response to them. A clinician who is internally focused upon 'the process' and the linear progression from beginning, through intervention and towards completion of the interaction, will inevitably fail to impact upon a child's experience.

It is fair to say that there is an art to this. Our ability to utilise these techniques effectively improves with practice. Additionally, the nature of the interaction is dynamic. It evolves and changes in real time.

5.4 Obstacles and Opportunities in a Child's Mindset

It is worth noting that many children attending for a medical intervention will ignore the attending clinician. The mechanism underpinning this pattern of behaviour represents one of a child's greatest strengths. If they refuse to engage with you, they can pretend you don't exist, and if you don't exist, then the intervention they are anxious about is not taking place. If they withdraw from their surroundings completely, then perhaps in their reality, they are no longer even in the hospital. This grants us some understanding of what we are up against in attempting to reach a child who has 'locked us out'. It will take something different to solve.

Fortunately for us and perhaps one of the reasons we elect to work with children, is that they have powerful imperatives when it comes to being inquisitive, fascination with all that is new, a celebration of humour, interest in games, engagement with technology, natural aptitude for fantasy and many more. In order to reach a child who has withdrawn into their own tailored reality, engaging them by triggering one such imperative can generate a 'point of entry', a means to reach them.

5.5 Strategies

The following strategies are taken from a broad range of specialties. The research and peer reviewed publications outlining these techniques is presented and examples of how and when they might be deployed in clinical practice illustrated where appropriate. Strategies appraised in this section include:

- EVT – Expectancy Violations Theory
- Touch – haptics
- Confusion/overload
- Incongruent behaviour
- Alternative point of entry
- Challenging negative frameworks and valence optimisation
- Tag-team talking
- Humour
- Distraction
- Yes Set
- The bind – an illusion of choice
- Tension/release
- Pseudo-orientation
- Validation
- Cognitive appraisal – understanding what and why
- Implied rapport
- Successive approximation
- Guided imagery and storytelling
- Hypnosis
- Magic
- Decompression

5.5.1 Expectancy Violations Theory (EVT) IF RB CS

Expectancy Violations Theory was described by Judee Burgoon (34, 70, 71). The theory was described as part of an attempt to understand observed effects of violations of personal space during social interaction. The core principles of this theory relevant to the management of PIA are:

- Unexpected behaviour causes arousal and compulsion to cognitively appraise the unexpected behaviour with subsequent evaluation to either a positive or negative valence.
- Expectancy is dictated by socially accepted norms, the valence or 'rewardingness' of the violator and finally the circumstances including context and physical elements of the environment including space.
- A positive valence or 'rewardingness' of an individual depends on the observer's perception of the violator's ability to reward or punish them either literally or indirectly in the form of social and intellectually reward attributed by association with an individual who is attractive, has status or power.
- The violation itself can have positive or negative valence depending on the appraisal of the individual experiencing it. Violations that are ambiguous are likely to be perceived as positive if the perpetrator has positive valence.
- The magnitude of the violation has an influence.
- A positive violation committed by a perpetrator with positive valence will have a greater and more positive influence on communication outcome than a positive

confirmation – an interaction where the perpetrator has positive valence and behaves as they are expected to – so confirming expectations.

- Extreme proximity is perceived as aversive.
- The more rewarding a perpetrator is perceived to be, the closer they are allowed to get before aversion is perceived.
- Arousal caused by violations can be on a cognitive level where you are mentally aware of the violation or on a physical level. This is important when appraising the effect of touch.
- Arousal level reaches a point where less attention is paid to the message being communicated and more to the source of arousal.
- The concept of 'threat threshold' refers to the point at which threat is perceived. Those who are anxious are more easily aroused and to a greater extent by a lesser degree of violation than those who are not.

So, what is the relevance of this in the management of PIA?

- An expectancy violation can be intentionally deployed to cause arousal, command attention and an external focus, which disrupts the characteristic internal focus associated with anxiety and forces an external re-evaluation.
- The period of external re-evaluation generated by an expectancy violation offers an opportunity to connect with the child, build rapport and implement coping strategies.
- Expectancy violation offers a means to further positively enhance the valence a clinician may already possess due to their perceived status and influence.

As we can see, this technique offers a unique opportunity to disrupt negative processes associated with anxiety and significantly enhance the potency of therapeutic connection in any management strategy.

An example of an expectancy violation that you as a clinician might employ would be to deliberately invade the child's personal space by putting your foot next to the child's foot, with the excuse of admiring their shoes and to see if their shoes would fit your foot. This simultaneously braids the violation with an excuse for executing it, rapport building and humour.

The use of expectancy violations is subtle yet very powerful. As Burgoon showed, it explains some of the idiosyncrasies of social interaction we see, in particular those regarding proxemics, although it applies to many strategies we employ, and offers us a means to significantly enhance and optimise our management of PIA.

5.5.2 Touch: Haptics IF RB

Touch can be utilised as an expectancy violation. It creates arousal, an external focus and re-appraisal. Additionally, the use of contact in the form of light touch has been shown to increase compliance (72–74).

With this in mind, touch deployed under the right circumstances and in the right way, is an effective technique in management of PIA. Naturally, there will be times where this technique is appropriate and times where it would represent an expectancy violation of such magnitude and negativity that it would be inappropriate and counterproductive.

The key to successful deployment of touch to enhance anxiety management is context. If the clinical context is such that touch would be part of the process then it can be safely deployed. In the absence of such a context, it may be generated by engaging the child in a process that involves physical contact. An example might be asking a child to grab your hand and help pull you up from your seat, with the excuse that you played sport with your own children at the weekend and are still a bit sore.

Why might touch have such a positive influence on rapport building and compliance? It may be that making physical contact, an activity normally reserved for those closest and most trusted, sub-consciously implies and confers equivalent status or valence to the stranger. More detailed discussion of proximity and its influence in communication can be found in the later section on proxemics.

5.5.3 Confusion/Overload IF ⟨cs⟩

There is an element of confusion in many advanced management techniques. This stems from its potency as a means to disrupt internal focus by commanding attention and generate an intense external focus facilitating re-evaluation of the situation. This creates an opportunity for the clinician to reach the child and establish a therapeutic connection through which they may harvest positive resources, build rapport, address concerns and deploy effective coping strategies.

The command of attention associated with confusion is driven by the unpleasant state of dissonance it elicits. Additionally, the more confused an individual becomes, the more dissonance they experience and the more desperate they will be to re-establish the status quo. If the confusion persists despite all attempts at re-orientation, eventually the need for resolution becomes so overwhelmingly powerful that the individual will accept *any* half decent explanation to make sense of things, no matter how irrational or illogical it might be. Under these circumstances the child has reached a point of overload at which they tend towards increased compliance and being hyper-suggestable, both of which will enhance the effectiveness of any anxiety management strategy deployed.

The simplest conversational approach to generate confusion is by establishing overload. This can be achieved by deploying a flight of ideas approach in verbal communication, on a subject that is engaging and humorous, while rapidly switching between topics with little more than an abstract connection between them. The novelty and humour deployed will gain the child's attention and the challenge of establishing connections between topics will ensure this attention does not waver. Eventually, the volume and complexity of associations are such that the child's capacity to make sense of the dialogue is exceeded, overload will have been achieved, the process of disruption, re-focusing and re-evaluation will have been triggered, and a tendency towards increased compliance and a hyper-suggestable state will have been established (75, 76).

A more complex technique for establishing confusion through conversation is to utilise ambiguous statements and words that *sound* exactly the same but have different meanings. When written on paper you can see which word is being utilised as they are spelt completely differently such as 'four' and 'for'. This is known as phonological ambiguity. For a listener to establish the meaning of sentences constructed in this manner, they must appraise each word in relation to the others as well as each sentence in relation to the overall context of the conversation. Naturally, this requires intense concentration and external focus. As such, intentionally deploying phonological ambiguity can be used to trigger the process of disruption, re-focusing and re-evaluation as part of an anxiety management strategy.

An example of this approach might be:

So, you like football?

Which club do you *support*?

Ah. I was watching a tournament they were in the other day.

They *calmly* won one 2-1 then drew one 2-2 too.

Easily went 3-1 two minutes into the next two.

Safely securing 1 4-1 and 2-1 for two more.

They were *SO relaxed*.

The opposition goal ate eight too for four games to win.

And the funny thing was they had two mascots in a tutu too.

In this example phonological ambiguity has been used in conversation regarding an interest in football with a view to generating confusion. An additional layer of therapeutic content has been braided into the final text in the form of positive suggestions, highlighted in italics. The intention would be to subtly exaggerate the delivery of the text in italics by altering the cadence, intonation or volume of speech. This has the potential to offer additional therapeutic content if a hyper-suggestable state has been achieved in addition to confusion.

In summary, we can see that confusion is an extremely effective tool in the management of anxiety. The more complex approaches to generating confusion can be challenging to design and deploy; however some may find them particularly useful and the process of designing and managing such interactions exceptionally rewarding.

It is worth noting that the simpler method for generating confusion can be effective for all ages, developmental stages and extremes of anxiety. However, the more complex form may be better suited and effective in children who are able and motivated to engage in the challenge the technique presents. Such children are more likely older children, at a more advanced stage of cognitive development and experiencing anxiety of mild or moderate intensity.

5.5.4 Incongruent Behaviour IF

Incongruent behaviour utilises an element of both confusion and expectancy violation. The child's preconceptions with regards to what clinicians are, what they should be and how they ought to behave will significantly influence their expectations with regards to hospital interactions. This grants an opportunity if we act and behave in a manner that overtly challenges these preconceptions. Deploying unexpected, unusual, odd yet amusing or novel behaviour will cause confusion and violate an expectancy. This will disrupt internal focus by commanding attention and generate an external focus so that re-evaluation of the situation can occur. This efficiently establishes a conduit through which a therapeutic connection may be established and coping strategies deployed.

The simplest of examples of this technique might be to walk into the patient's room and immediately sit on the floor. Essentially, any behaviour that departs from the stereotypical pattern of behaviour that a professional and gravely serious clinician could reasonably be expected to use, will do. Naturally, behaviour can be far more amusing and incongruent than this, although one should be aware of the limits within which behaviour remains clinically and socially acceptable.

5.5.5 Alternative Point of Entry IF RB

This strategy promotes adopting an unconventional manner when interacting with a child at the time of first contact. A conventional approach would be to engage in medical processing at the outset. Adopting an alternative point of entry involves setting the child, their interests and rapport building as the primary focus. Such an approach sends a powerful therapeutic message, that the child is of paramount importance, not the medical process. In addition, deviating from expected behaviour causes confusion which attracts attention and disrupts *internal* focus by commanding an external re-evaluation of the situation. This period of re-evaluation generates an opportunity to engage the child and build rapport by utilising known resources and those that may be observed in the moment such as pictures on the T-shirt they are wearing, toys they are holding or engaging them through any activity they are currently engaged in.

Engagement in an all-consuming activity is one of the most commonly encountered dysfunctional coping strategies deployed by anxious children. Although these activities or props create a barrier to connection and communication, it is possible to integrate them within an anxiety management strategy by utilising them as a means to reach and connect with the child. For example, a child hiding behind an electronic device may be intentionally deploying it as distraction, a physical barrier for protection, an excuse for avoiding eye contact and a means to prevent conversation. However, by expressing credible interest in the activity or game being played and an inquisitive nature, the clinician can convert what might be perceived by some as an insurmountable obstacle, into *the* means to reach and establish therapeutic connection with the child. Once this connection has been established, the child's interests can be harvested, genuine rapport can evolve, concerns can be established and coping strategies deployed.

Examples of utilising other visible resources might include engaging the child through an interest in football evidenced by a team shirt they are wearing or chatting about a film they are watching. One of the most disarming approaches is enthusiastically requesting an explanation about what they are doing or watching. What could be better than someone taking an interest in what *you* are interested in and asking for your expert opinion?

5.5.6 Challenging Negative Preconceptions ⓇⒷ IF

Many children will come to hospital with negative preconceptions regarding clinicians. This may simply represent a fear of strangers, or it may be the consequence of past negative experiences. Under such circumstances, a child may perceive a clinician as a negative entity, inhuman in many respects, simply an 'it' to be feared as opposed to a person they have never met before. An effective strategy to challenge this type of negative perception is to find an opportunity to share information that illustrates your humanity. This would include talking about being a father or mother and your own children if you have any, discussing your pets, asking if they have any and if they do, asking for details. Pictures and videos kept on your phone are particularly useful to engage, occupy and distract them. Alternatives include talking about your interests or activities away from the workplace and any element of non-medical existence. You may share interests allowing an exchange of views. Sharing information in this way allows the child to see you as a person, like them. You become a 'who' rather than a 'what' and by challenging *these* negative assumptions, you pose the question whether all of their preconceptions might be questionable. At the very least, you generate a platform for therapeutic connection and an opportunity to build rapport.

It is worth acknowledging that we may not know which child has established negative preconceptions and which does not. As such, we should employ this strategy for all children with a view to significantly contributing to the rapport building process, and addressing negative expectation where they exist.

5.5.7 Tag-Team Talking IF CS

This advanced technique commands external focus at the same time as deploying a coping strategy in the form of distraction. It involves the braiding of two separate lines of verbal communication run in parallel. One is always the linear clinical process of moving from point A to point B in getting the medical job done, for example taking a history, or check-in through to intervention. The other is a completely medically unrelated conversation that ideally commands the child's attention through its novelty, abstract content, relevance to the child, utilisation of the child's resources and/or deployment of any of the other coping strategies. Confusion, humour and magic would be excellent choices in this setting.

An illustration would be braiding a linear sequence of routine medical questions with a conversation about the child's favourite television program, so that they run in parallel. By bouncing from one step in the routine process, to the completely unrelated non-medical subject, then back again to the medical and so on, the child and parent must concentrate hard to follow both lines of conversation which commands an external focus at the same time as completing the task at hand. If the non-medical element is humorous or integrates incongruent entertaining behaviour then the child's natural tendency to be inquisitive and fun-loving will be engaged. This will further enhance rapport and represent a coping strategy by connecting with positive resources and offering distraction through engagement in the task.

In itself, this approach can be seen as a compound strategy as it braids elements of incongruent behaviour, expectancy violation, confusion, distraction and humour within a single interaction, all in parallel. In understanding this technique, we should note two things. First, as with many techniques, in order for it to be successful, the clinician must be focused, have the capacity to follow their own train of thought and maintain a view of how and what they are trying to achieve throughout. Second is the acknowledgement that most anxiety management strategies are delivered covertly and consist of complex compound strategies generated by braiding multiple techniques. Interventions of this nature, complex yet unremarkable and undetectable, represent the gold standard in anxiety management. They deliver maximal influence while generating minimal resistance by evading detection.

5.5.8 Humour CS

We are all familiar with humour. It is perhaps one of the most, if not *the* most familiar pastime and is linked to a set of positive conditioned responses and emotions. As such, braiding humour into our working practice is one of the easiest and most effective ways we can deploy positive conditioned behaviour patterns as part of any management strategy.

Some of us are more comfortable than others when wielding humour. Some of us are naturally funny and can deliver a joke well. For those who struggle, it can be argued the absence of this natural ability offers an opportunity as long as the individual concerned can understand how to make the most of it. Many comedians have based their whole career around being serious and lacking humour. Their 'straightness' creates a harsher clearer backdrop to the humour making it more obvious and, in many respects, funnier. For those who really struggle to remember a joke, ask the child if they know one. When a child remembers a joke, it will be one that *they* thought was funny which means it is guaranteed to connect with positive resources specific to them.

One example of a simple approach to humour that anyone can deploy would be to add a title to the child's name within the formal procedure of checking consent. This particular example is an incredibly effective way to diffuse tension that tends to peak just prior to any medical intervention. It may be most effective in the younger age groups but not exclusively so.

Finally, a word of caution should complete any comment on the use of humour in a clinical setting. It must be recognised that any attempt at humour needs to be appropriate in terms of the situation, content, political correctness and age of the child. Having said this, when granted an opportunity, nothing will prevent some children sharing grossly inappropriate jokes, much to the embarrassment of their parents.

5.5.9 Distraction IF CS

We have all encountered distraction as an anxiety management technique. It disrupts internal focus by engaging the child in an external process and it represents a coping strategy when the source of distraction engages the child with their own positive resources.

Distraction will most likely succeed when a child is motivated to engage in the process, such as in the presence of rapport, if an approach is novel, appeals to them and commands their attention, or if it is familiar to them and linked with a pre-conditioned positive response such as their favourite film, games or music. They must be interested in the form of distraction deployed. For example, asking a 6-year-old child to join you looking at today's news is less likely to work than getting them to play a game of their choice on an electronic device. In this age of technology and the overwhelming move towards the use of electronic devices, the use of phones, tablets and multimedia storage devices has become familiar. As such, these will undoubtedly offer a means to access preconditioned positive resources for most children. Equally, as these devices become commonplace, other media may become novel and engaging as an alternative resource to engage and distract.

For distraction to be successful, we should utilise a single clear process to avoid generating confusion, and deliver this in a calm, relaxed, unhurried manner. Sadly, we have all witnessed the antithesis of this, when multiple individuals, all of whom appear anxious and agitated themselves, fight each other for a child's attention as they simultaneously seek to deliver their own chosen form of distraction. Unfortunately, although such behaviour stems from good intentions, it will inevitably lead to confusion and an increased level of anxiety for the child. In such situations the clinician should, where possible, calmly seek to gain the attention of the individuals involved, establish control and impose a clear direction with regards to any distraction being deployed.

It is worth noting, there are a small number of children who may perceive an attempt at distraction as an attempt at deception. These children commonly have past negative experiences that have undermined rapport and their trust in those that are caring for them. As a direct consequence, they are more likely to resist overt attempts at gaining compliance and will often refuse to engage with anxiety management strategies. Under these circumstances, it is worth seeking input from practitioners experienced in elective therapeutic behaviour modification techniques with a view to improving the child's future experiences, optimise the chances of successful medical intervention and most importantly, avoid causing additional psychological trauma.

5.5.10 Yes Set CS RB

The Yes Set is a technique first described by Erickson and Rossi, for overcoming resistance to suggestion delivered as part of a hypnotherapeutic intervention (77, 78). Despite originating from the field of speaking therapies, the technique has been utilised in everyday life as a means to enhance compliance by braiding it with regular non-therapeutic verbal communication. An example of such practice comes from the field of marketing where it is used in an attempt to increase the success rate of sales pitches.

The technique hinges upon making a series of statements, directed at the recipient, that are obviously true or correct. This is then followed by the statement with which compliance is being sought. The sequence of truisms builds up a patterned response in the listener. As they appraise the statements, whether answering or just listening, they build up a sequence of responses in the affirmative, a Yes Set. This repetitive sequence, where every response is a 'yes', generates a degree of pressure for the listener to maintain the harmony by continuing the series with another 'yes', rather than an incongruous and disruptive 'no'.

This is such a simple technique that anyone can use it and in any situation. It is relatively easy to think of a sequence of statements or questions that will gain an affirmative response even in a clinical setting. Using this type of sequence as a prelude to the question we want to be answered with a 'yes', will increase the likelihood of success.

It is worth commenting on states of consciousness and receptivity to suggestion. Many hypnotherapeutic techniques, like the Yes Set, can be used to great effect in everyday interaction in the form of conversational suggestion. The potency of these techniques in anxiety management stems from the associated hyper-suggestible state. It is a mistake to think of the awake state and altered state of consciousness as binary, that we exist in one or the other as discrete entities. In reality, we are in neither one nor the other. What we define as consciousness encompasses all states as a dynamic and fluid reality within which we shift continuously throughout the day. As such, the degree to which our 'state' makes us more or less receptive to influence and suggestion is in continuous flux.

Recognising and accepting this fluidity of consciousness and the increased sensitivity to suggestion anxiety bestows on a child, grants an opportunity to appreciate and utilise the powerful influence conversational suggestion delivers, when deployed as part of an anxiety management strategy. Conversational suggestion is discussed in greater detail in section 4.7.

5.5.11 The Bind: An Illusion of Choice ⓒⓢ

Children have a tendency towards resistance. Anxious children certainly do. As such, the ability to manage or preferably circumvent resistance is essential for clinicians managing the anxious child. Any attempt to manage directly and overtly is, by definition, almost certain to precipitate further resistance.

One technique that allows effective management is the bind. This is such a simple technique and for those with children of their own, it is a technique they will recognise and often deploy at home.

From Erickson and Rossi (78) – 'A *bind* offers a patient a free, conscious choice between two or more alternatives. Whichever choice is made, however, leads the patient in the same therapeutic direction.' Yapko refers to The Bind as a bind of comparable alternatives in *Trancework*, p. 258 (79).

In principle, it is giving the patient the illusion of choice by allowing them to choose between two alternatives. However, both options result in the exact same and desired outcome.

An example taken from an anaesthetic interaction might be to ask a child, 'Would you like to sit on your parent's lap or the trolley to go to sleep'? The child will appreciate being given a choice rather than told what to do, but whichever option they go for, they will be accepting that they are going to sleep. This is simple, yet often effective.

5.5.12 Tension/Release IF cs

To use this technique the clinician deliberately creates tension within the child, then releases it. By generating tension then releasing it, a sense of relaxation is both generated and accentuated.

An example of this might be to very seriously, as part of the medical dialogue, state that you wish to check some very important information. Once the child registers this and awaits any further questions with a heightened sense of expectancy, the clinician might release the tension by asking a humorous question such as – 'How big do you think my parrot's hands are'? This creates and then relieves tension at the same time as utilising humour to form the abstract image of a parrot with hands.

5.5.13 Pseudo-orientation cs

Pseudo-orientation refers explicitly to a hypnotherapeutic technique whereby a subject is asked to imagine that they can travel forward in time to a point where they have completed the task they are struggling with. They are then asked to describe how they might have had to change to achieve what currently appears unachievable. Additionally, they are asked about any alterations in their perspective, resources they would have needed to find, and any lessons they may have learned as a consequence. They are then asked to imagine travelling back to the present day, bringing with them all of the abilities, changes and resources they had imagined as part of this exercise. They are asked to visualise themselves as that individual, now, here in the present (80).

The primary purpose of this approach is to get the subject to consider the possibility that they might actually be able to achieve what they have seen as impossible. The secondary purpose is to get them to consider the changes required to complete the task and how they will benefit when they do. As such the exercise creates belief in their ability to achieve, understanding of what might be required to do so, acceptance that they possess the resources that will be needed and an understanding of the benefits they will appreciate as a direct consequence. This latter aspect is very important as it generates motivation which in turn increases compliance.

This technique is very useful as a tool used in elective anxiety management which is discussed in a later section. A more simplistic version would be to ask the child to imagine and talk about just the benefits they will gain if they complete the task.

5.5.14 Validation RB cs

Validation in the context of anxiety management means to recognise and validate the feelings, thoughts, behaviour and experiences of the child. Parents and those attempting to support an anxious child often feel helpless, yet wish to resolve the child's anxiety. In attempting to do so, they may inadvertently *in*-validate the feelings, thoughts, behaviour and experiences of the child affected.

To illustrate, when an child says; 'I am anxious', the parent may reply: 'You're alright', 'It's OK', or 'It's all fine'. When this interaction is analysed literally, the child is indicating that they are *not* OK, yet the parent's reply indicates that in their opinion nothing is wrong and that the child is, in fact, just fine. Such an interaction may be the product of functional management strategies for everyday existence such as when a child grazes their knee during play. Making light of challenging or painful experiences that are common in everyday life promotes functional proportionate evaluation and responses. However, when this same strategy is applied in a situation that is completely out of the norm and extremely distressing, the child fails to gain the reassurance they so desperately need. Additionally, failure to validate the child's reality sends an implied message that the parent does not feel there is a problem. As a consequence, they are perceived as lacking empathy and may be discounted as a source of support. If this happens, it must be incredibly frustrating and generates a sense of abandonment and loneliness in the child. Naturally, few parents would intentionally cause distress or fail to offer support, but it is often seen in the manner described above, and when this happens it will almost certainly make the child's anxiety worse.

It has been shown that validation of a child's experience, particularly if they tend to experience strong emotions, reduces the magnitude of their responses and helps them manage their feelings more effectively (81). Validation in behaviour therapy, specifically related to psychotherapy for the treatment of suicidal behaviour, was defined by Marsha Linehan as:

> The essence of validation is this. The therapist communicates to the client that her responses make sense and are understandable within her current life context or situation. The therapist actively accepts the client and communicates this acceptance to the client. The therapist takes the client's responses seriously and does not discount or trivialize them. Validation strategies require the therapist to search for, recognize and reflect to the client the validity inherent in her response to events (82).

In terms of managing PIA, it is important for us to recognise a child's experiences and show them we understand and appreciate how they feel and why. This helps to manage and reduce anxiety, enhances rapport building and maintains a conduit for therapeutic intervention and support. From the child's perspective, if we understand how they feel then we have taken the first step towards being able to help them.

So, from a practical standpoint, tell the child you understand how they feel. You may tell them that it's normal and unsurprising that in this situation they might feel anxious and that in many respects if they didn't feel this way it would be a bit odd. Medical interventions are generally an unusual occurrence rather than a regular experience and will nearly always generate some level of anxiety or apprehension. Having validated the child's reality and enhanced rapport, you will have created an opportunity to implement a coping strategy and offer support.

5.5.15 Cognitive Appraisal ◈

This is a form of validation in that the clinician clearly illustrates that they understand and accept the child's reality. In addition, they will aim to help the child understand and gain perspective on their feelings and any physiological changes that may be taking place.

Children who display significant general anxiety or PIA can develop phobic or freeze–flight–fight responses that are triggered in a hospital environment. When this happens and a sense of panic sets in, the physiological responses and changes the child experiences can terrify them. They may feel there is something physically wrong, that the changes are part of some physical illness or that they should be able to control themselves but can't. If left unchecked, such processes will reinforce themselves each time the child is exposed to the anxiogenic stimulus.

Those who experience extreme anxiety or phobic responses will require elective intervention by a specialist multidisciplinary team (MDT). For the many children who experience mild or intermediate levels of panic, explaining how and why the anxiety process works and helping them understand that any associated physiological changes are natural, protective and nothing to fear, is cognitive therapy delivered in the acute setting. If the child has a better understanding of their own reality, it can become less frightening. Helping them realise there is nothing wrong with them psychologically or physically and that they are not expected to be able to control the physical changes taking place, completes this process of cognitive reframing. At this point the conditions in which an anxious child can calm down and re-connect with those supporting them will have been generated.

An example of how this cognitive appraisal might be achieved would be to tell the child you understand how they feel, then explain how their ongoing response is exactly like a deer chased by a lion which they may have seen on wildlife programmes on TV. The response and physiology of the deer allows them to react quickly and protect themselves. An animal that experiences a threat like this will take note of the environment in which it happens and the next time they notice they are in a similar environment the same protective systems will be activated in case the same thing happens again. By explaining in this manner the child will be able to appreciate their own response is a normal protective mechanism triggered by being in a strange place or interventions they may feel anxious about.

This is such a simple technique, yet its influence as part of an anxiety management strategy will be significant.

5.5.16 Successive Approximation CS

Successive approximation involves taking any process of medical intervention that is generating significant anxiety, and breaking it up into smaller steps that the child is able to cope with. The success of this strategy is dependent on reducing the level of anxiogenic stimuli at any one point in time to one the child can cope with.

An example might be for a child having a cannula inserted on the ward prior to attending the theatre suite for surgery. This will separate the anxiety generated by cannulation from anxiety that may be generated by the rest of the journey. This technique is probably one of the most commonly deployed techniques in clinical practice.

5.5.17 Guided Imagery and Storytelling CS IF

Guided imagery utilises verbal suggestion or commentary to stimulate sensory perception which leads to the accessing of positive resources in the form of memories, thoughts, feelings and sensations. This may take the form of storytelling, describing real or imaginary experiences that are general in nature or specific to the person engaged in the imagery. The goal of the process is to reduce stress, anxiety and negative emotions in order to attain a positive harmonious mental state.

In clinical practice it is possible to deploy guided imagery to maintain disruption of internal focus characteristic of the anxiety state while additionally accessing positive resources as a coping strategy. Accessing these positive resources has been shown to help patients manage anxiety and improve clinical outcome after an intervention (83–86).

When deploying guided imagery, suggestions should be deployed in a manner that stimulates the full range of senses in order to generate stimuli that are as rich and detailed as possible. Many individuals will have a dominant sensory system that they favour when formulating memories or cataloguing experiences. If you ask a person to access a memory, then describe it to you, they will represent what they remember and experienced preferentially in terms of this dominant or primary representation system – for example dominantly what they see or hear. If you know what a person's primary representation system is, then you can tailor your suggestions to target this system for that individual.

For many children, the simple act of asking them to imagine they are on the beach or riding their bike/horse, or tucked up safe in their bed at night while describing the experience in detail, will be enough to engage and distract them at the same time as accessing positive resources and the positive state that will come as a consequence.

An example of effective imagery for a child would be talking to them about being warm in the sun at the beach while a light breeze keeps them cool. Being tired after playing in the sea, they decide to lie down on a towel or sunbed to get some rest. They might decide to shut their eyes just for a little while, to rest them, and listen to the waves on the sand. As they listen they realise the waves come in threes. The first wave is louder and long, the second is gentler and a bit shorter and the third of the trio is somewhere in-between ... then they start again. They may be aware of the sound of seagulls and children playing while the wind gently rustles the grass or trees.

Storytelling is a variant of this skillset. The story can be generic or preferably it should be specifically tailored to include things or characters the child is interested in. Braiding personalised elements into the story such as their favourite characters or the hobbies they are interested in, enhances motivation to engage with the story and should enhance the effectiveness of the suggestions it contains. Effective stories will incorporate significant therapeutic content in the form of reassuring, relaxing and supportive suggestions. Finally, there is always the opportunity in storytelling to braid other coping strategies into the process such as humour with a view to maximising the therapeutic effect.

In Yapko's hypnotherapy textbook *Trancework* (79) he gives an excellent description of how to construct a therapeutic intervention. His approach to constructing therapy applies to storytelling and many other interventions. First, you should define the problem that needs addressing, then define the resources the client will need to address the problem. Once this has been done you need to establish which of these resources they already have and finally to design an intervention with a view to delivering and installing the resources that are missing. This is an outstandingly simple yet comprehensive framework for any planned intervention.

5.5.18 Hypnosis IF RB CS

In 1892 The British Medical Association commissioned a group of medical experts to evaluate the use of hypnosis in medical practice. Later that year they published their report in the *British Medical Journal* confirming, among other things, that the hypnosis was real, and the hypnotic state was indeed genuine (87).

In 1953 the Psychological Medicine Group of The BMA set up a subcommittee to examine the use of hypnosis in medical practice. Their report, published in The *BMJ* on 23 April 1955, made it clear that they agreed with the findings published in 1892.

Additionally, they commended the foresight of the 1892 committee and among other pertinent comments, stated the following:

> In addition to the treatment of psychiatric disabilities, there is a place for hypnotism in the production of anaesthesia or analgesia for surgical and dental operations, and in suitable subjects it is an effective method of relieving pain in childbirth without altering the normal course of labour.
>
> It is recommended that a description of hypnotism and its therapeutic possibilities, limitations, and dangers should be given to medical undergraduates during their psychiatric course.
>
> Instruction in the clinical use of hypnotism should be given to all medical postgraduates training as specialists in psychological medicine and possibly, say, to trainee anaesthetists and obstetricians, so that they will understand its indications and practical applications (88).

Some three years after this report was published, The American Medical Association commissioned their own report and lent their full support to the position adopted by the BMA (89).

Current research utilising functional MRI supports these views and recommendations in proving unequivocally that the hypnotic trance is a real and discrete state evidenced by characteristic neurophysiological activity (90). Additionally, there is clear evidence that hypnosis can reduce pain and anxiety in children undergoing medical interventions (91–95), and enhance immune function (96).

In considering the committee reports from 1892, 1955 and 1958, along with research evidence on the subject, it is difficult to argue *against* providing medical undergraduates with an understanding of hypnosis and training in its use. These reports and current research findings support the integration of hypnosis and hypnotherapy into mainstream practice.

Hypnosis is a powerful tool for the management of PIA. It can be used in both the elective and emergent setting, either in a formal structured approach or by utilising conversational suggestion. Elective management of PIA and conversational suggestion are discussed in separate sections. Hypnosis requires no tools, just a trained individual. Hypnotic trance can be established with or without speech. An example of a trance phenomenon encountered in everyday existence, that is established without verbal input, would be time distortion experienced on long journeys when an individual 'zones out' during the trip. This is often referred to as 'highway hypnosis' and is one experienced while in an altered state of consciousness.

In coming to understand hypnosis and its clinical value, we must fully appreciate the concept of altered states. As mentioned earlier, state does not exist in binary. Our state should not be seen as altered or not altered. In reality, our state is dynamic and in continuous flux. In a similar manner, we should not think of ourselves or others as hypnotised and suggestable or not. We are all open to suggestion at any time. In the same manner, a child can transition to a state of anxiety, and therefore can easily transition back out again with appropriate support.

Techniques including hypnotic suggestion, that facilitate movement from one aspect of state to another, can be deployed covertly to evade detection and prevent resistance. They can be braided into patterns of normal behaviour and communication, offering an approach perfectly suited to the management of PIA. When one considers this and the fact children are generically suggestable, with anxiety further enhancing this characteristic, failing to deploy such techniques including hypnosis in the management of PIA would be to miss a significant opportunity.

A full explanation of the process of hypnosis is beyond the scope of this section. As referenced earlier, Yapko's *Trancework* (79) offers an excellent introduction to the subject, but there are many others. An excellent account of hypnosis and suggestion, its use and misuse can be found in Robert Temple's *Open to Suggestion* (97). Even a limited understanding of the hypnotic process will allow a clinician to dovetail this form of communication into conversation or to implement the formal process of hypnotic induction, establish a trance, deepen this trance with a view to reducing fear and anxiety, then redirect the child to a more acceptable state. As has been established, there may be an opportunity to deliver additional therapeutic benefit once a trance state has been established.

An example of braiding hypnosis into everyday practice would be the use of a formal hypnotic approach prior to taking bloods or inserting a cannula on the ward. This could be achieved by simply asking the child to close their eyes and taking them through a relaxation exercise, then deepening the sense of relaxation and suggesting that the area of skin where venepuncture will take place is numb. Following such a suggestion and after the intervention has taken place, the clinician should always suggest the return of all sensation to normal. Whenever suggestion or formal hypnosis is deployed there will be an opportunity to reinforce a general sense of wellbeing and confidence as a generically therapeutic strategy, prior to finalising the process.

In summary, hypnosis is real, clinically effective and easy to deploy. It is free, portable and can be tailored for use in any situation instantaneously. Why wouldn't we use it?

5.5.19 Magic IF CS

A belief in magic is one of the superpowers all children possess! The others include eternal optimism, an infinitely powerful imagination and inexhaustible supplies of forgiveness.

There are many complex and advanced magic techniques. That said, allied to a child's inexhaustible belief, even the simplest of magic tricks represents a powerful adjunct in the management of PIA. Learning to do a simple coin trick through sleight-of-hand will deliver a significant return on your investment of time and effort. The inability of a child to ignore a magic trick almost guarantees disruption of any internal focus, accessing of more positive resources and the generation of an opportunity to implement additional coping strategies. You can even use these skills to engage and connect with children by showing them how the trick is done and teaching them to perform the trick themselves.

5.5.20 Decompression CS RB

This last technique couldn't be simpler. Never underestimate the power of 'backing off'. To just STOP. Continuing an attempt to move a process of intervention forward when it is precipitating significant and escalating anxiety makes no sense. Failure to defuse the situation will more than likely reinforce whatever process has been established in terms of conditioned responses, inflict additional psychological damage and further undermine the relationship with parent and clinician.

In this situation, adopting the opposite approach is likely to achieve the diametrically opposite effect. It avoids reinforcement of the conditioned response, avoids inflicting additional trauma and not only avoids further undermining the relationship with parent and clinician, but it actually enhances it. By showing a child we are listening, that we understand the consequences of their current reality and that no one is going to physically enforce compliance, we regain or start to regain their trust. This approach also offers an opportunity to re-evaluate the situation and adopt an alternate management strategy. An alternate approach might simply be letting the child calm down and looking to deploy sedation to assist in the process. Alternatively, it may involve a formal elective management strategy delivered by an MDT or something in-between these two extremes.

Many children have underlying and often complex issues that are extremely difficult to manage without elective intervention and a carefully tailored management strategy being implemented. Attempting to cobble something together in an acute setting, under less than ideal circumstances may be necessary as the very last resort, when a delay to intervention is potentially life-threatening. However, the risks of causing further psychological damage are significant.

So, be ready to stop when it is appropriate. Maintaining a perspective from which effective evaluation of the situation is possible will protect the relationships required to help an anxious child and avoid inflicting further unnecessary trauma.

Key Points

- There is no complete or fully comprehensive list of enhanced communication strategies, nor can there be.
- Management strategies are fluid, bespoke and must by nature maintain a fluidity in its true sense, morphing to fill any void they are designed to fill.
- Strategies must appear consistent or congruent with the apparent personality and nature of the clinician delivering them. As such, strategies that appear congruent and are effective will vary between clinicians.
- Deploying enhanced strategies in isolation, in the absence of congruent covert, overt verbal and non-verbal communication, consistent with optimal anxiety management, will likely have *minimal* impact upon a child's anxiety. An opportunity to optimally manage anxiety will be generated when *all* forms of communication align to signal non-threat, calm, control and are utilised to build rapport and trust.
- There are many ways to understand the effects of strategies upon their recipient. One way to categorise them is to group them in terms of their influence upon internal focus, rapport building or their ability to offer a coping strategy.
- Strategies that disrupt the internal focus characteristic of anxiety states, command external focus and generate an opportunity to 'reach' the child.
- Reaching and connecting with a child makes them accessible. It is then up to the clinician to offer an anxiety management strategy.
- Communication and enhanced communication techniques may appear complex and their utilisation daunting; however, it should be acknowledged that we have all been communicating on multiple levels, every second of each day, for the entirety of our lives. As such, each and every one of us is an expert in communication.
- Our capacity to appropriately and effectively select, deploy and continuously re-evaluate management strategies in real time must match the dynamism and fluidity of the behaviour we are seeking to manage.
- Becoming comfortable and confident when optimising communication and deploying enhanced strategies takes time. We all start with the simplest techniques and build upon these. Anything we choose to try has merit and will make a difference. As we become

more confident and adept, the complexity and refinement of the patterns of communication we deploy will evolve to a point where such behaviour requires little if any conscious input, is 'invisible' to the observer and is extremely potent in terms of anxiety management.

- As our understanding of communication evolves, we will develop a full range of techniques. In any given situation, we can deploy these either in isolation or simultaneously and in parallel, with the most successful noted and adopted as an effective strategy while those that have little or no influence are abandoned.

Premedication

In a perfect world we would help all children develop effective coping strategies. This would empower them and allow them to manage their own anxieties independent of anyone or anything. However, this may not be possible due to the constraints of time or the child's capacity. Under such circumstances, premedication may offer an invaluable anxiety management strategy.

Examples of such situations include:

- When postponing an extremely anxious child's procedure, to allow an elective therapeutic intervention, is not an option.
- When a child is yet to reach a level of cognitive development that would allow effective coping strategies to be nurtured.
- If a child has been negatively conditioned following recurrent negative experiences, premedication may offer a means to manage interventions going forward by achieving an experience that is at worst, not negative and at best positive. If a series of interventions are managed in this way, it may be possible to help the child re-learn, to dismantle the conditioned negative response and replace it with a positive, functional pattern of ideation and behaviour.
- Lastly, premedication may be requested if it has been used successfully in the past or when it is selected as a preferred strategy going forward.

In essence, premedication can offer a strategy in and of itself, or a temporary solution until elective therapeutic intervention, targeting the development of coping strategies, can be delivered.

6.1 Acceptance/Refusal

Naturally, premedication is only an option if it is accepted as one. A small proportion of children refuse to take premeds. This may be due to the unpleasant taste of many agents. It is unfortunate that there has been little investment by the pharmaceutical industry in terms of seeking predication that is palatable.

Some children may refuse premedication if they fear losing or ceding control to those around them. Concerns of this nature are common when there is an absence of trust, lack of rapport, unfamiliar individuals are delivering care or if the child has been a victim of real or perceived deception in the past.

Premedication may be refused if a child was given a premed in the past to help manage overwhelming anxiety, it subsequently failed to achieve the desired outcome for whatever reason, yet the clinicians proceeded with the intervention anyway.

The experiential reality for the child living through such a sequence of events can be represented in the following way:

1. The child invests trust in those caring for them.
2. They take a premed on the basis they are promised it will reduce their anxiety and help them cope with the planned procedure.
3. The premed fails to deliver on this promise.
4. The child's trust in the clinicians is undermined.
5. The clinicians do not acknowledge the failure to achieve anxiolytic premedication which further undermines rapport and trust.
6. They then proceed with the planned intervention even though the child clearly communicates an extreme level of distress. This inflicts emotional trauma in addition to physical stress if restraint is deployed.
7. The clinicians' understanding of the child's concerns, the compassion they appeared to display and their promise to do everything possible to help the child are proven to be lies as far as the child is concerned.
8. Rapport and trust are critically undermined.

When one evaluates this process, it is difficult to imagine a more effective way to maximise psychological damage, undermine trust and discourage compliance in the future. Yet this happens. It requires little imagination to see that children who have experienced this may refuse premedication on the basis that taking it would mean they are agreeing to the exact same thing happening again. Accepting such treatment would likely represent a further insult to their emotional wellbeing, while refusing premeds in future may well be the last act of a child attempting to maintain their intellectual and emotional integrity.

If this pattern of behaviour, originally adopted as a temporising coping strategy, is reinforced and becomes entrenched, it will inevitably require expert elective intervention to dismantle. Once this process is completed, additional time will be required to generate coping strategies, regain trust and establish alternate functional patterns of behaviour that will support future successful medical interventions.

6.2 Snatching Defeat from the Jaws of Victory

On occasion a clinician may find the act of administering premedication generates as much if not greater anxiety than any planned intervention. Under such circumstances, the use of premedication as a management strategy should be re-evaluated. If anxiety is generated as the direct consequence of the process of administration, it may be possible to adjust this aspect of care allowing delivery of the medication uneventfully. If the child is actively resistant to premedication, such as described in the example above, careful consideration should precede any decision to adopt an approach utilising covert administration. Although it may succeed the first time, such an approach may further undermine trust and generate additional difficulties in the longer term. For example, following the covert use of a child's favourite drink to deliver a premed, if they later realise how they were tricked, they may refuse all drinks in similar situations in the future.

If the physical act of delivering a premed generates anxiety to the point the child becomes physically resistant, one has to question the benefit of this approach unless giving the premed successfully achieves anxiolysis and will cause less distress than proceeding without it. Naturally, elective input should be sought if at all feasible in this situation prior to any intervention. If the child is anxious, has limited capacity and an intervention is absolutely necessary, deploying a suitable number of staff in a coordinated manner and delivering premedication via the nasal or intramuscular route, in an attempt to reduce the time taken and coercion required to complete the process of administration, may minimise the psychological impact upon the child.

Lastly, when deploying more than one drug to achieve anxiolysis, it is worth considering the impact of delivering multiple premeds via different routes. If a child is to receive one drug nasally and a second into the buccal space which requires the active rubbing of the cheek or gum, the combined experience may generate unnecessary additional distress. Under such circumstances, if it's possible to deliver both agents via the same route, then this may be preferable.

6.3 Sedation Anxiolysis: Anxiety Dynamic

It is intuitive, yet worth highlighting, that successful premedication is a dynamic process weighing sedation anxiolysis against anxiety. As such, if a child is extremely agitated, to the point they are experiencing a full-blown freeze–flight–fight response, they will likely require a larger dose of premedication than a child who is relatively docile. A small subset of patients who experience the most extreme levels of anxiety may require premedication at doses exceeding the maximum recommended in standard protocols. If management of such children is to be effective, under exceptional and carefully considered circumstances, protocols will need to accommodate doses above and beyond the standard maximal limit. Naturally, particularly where administering outside standard protocols, patient safety must remain our first priority.

6.4 Organisation and Timing

Achieving optimal anxiolysis or sedation at exactly the right moment can be challenging. In addition to the considerations outlined above, if effective management of PIA is to be achieved, those prescribing and administering premedication must remain focused upon the child's needs, be willing to make exceptions with regards to standard protocols, communicate effectively and work together as one team. For surgical interventions, there may be a need for a 'holding area' within the theatre complex where premedication can be carefully timed and delays in the attendance for surgery minimised.

6.5 Agents

It is not the function of this text to present a detailed pharmacological account of the drugs at our disposal when seeking to deploy anxiolytic premedication. Commonly encountered drugs used in paediatric practice at this time include benzodiazepines mainly in the form of midazolam; alpha 2 agonists including dexmedetomidine and clonidine; opioids such as sufentanil, fentanyl and oral morphine; and ketamine, a phencyclidine derivative NMDA receptor antagonist. The therapeutic effect, patient tolerance and side effects vary according to the agent deployed and the route of delivery. This variety empowers clinicians to carefully select the agent and route of administration to suit the specific needs of each and every child. Unfortunately, although most clinicians and children tend to prefer the oral route of administration, most commonly available preparations are unpleasant to taste. As a consequence, they are often mixed with flavoured drinks that are selected by the recipient.

6.5.1 Midazolam

As a benzodiazepine, midazolam enhances the effect of gamma amino butyric acid in the central nervous system, generating anxiolysis, sedation and anterograde amnesia. The route of administration and dose for premedication includes oral: 0.5–0.75 mg/kg up to a maximum dose of 20 mg; buccal 0.3 mg/kg; nasal: 0.3 mg/kg; rectal: 0.5 mg/kg; and IV: 0.1 mg/kg. The most popular of these is the oral route, delivering an onset time of 10–20 minutes (98–100). One problem with midazolam is its bitter taste which can significantly and negatively influence patient satisfaction and ease of administration. Ozalin, a new preparation of midazolam, addresses this issue by incorporating inert excipient γ-cyclodextrin within the solution leading to the formation of inclusion complexes that enhance drug solubility and masks the bitter taste (101). Common side effects of midazolam include respiratory depression, particularly when administered in combination with an opioid or other respiratory depressant, paradoxical excitation or agitation and mucosal irritation when administered via the nasal route (102).

6.5.2 Clonidine

Clonidine is a mixed alpha receptor agonist with a predominant effect on alpha 2 receptors (103, 104). It delivers anxiolysis, sedation, enhanced analgesia and sympatholysis by activating alpha 2 receptors. Hypotension and bradycardia are generated by activation of alpha 1 receptors. The route of administration and dose as a premed include oral: 4–5 mics/kg; nasal: 2–4 mics/kg. It can also be administered IM, IV and PR although these routes are rarely utilised for premedication. Its longer onset time of 40–60 minutes can make timing of administration more challenging. Absence of paradoxical agitation and enhanced analgesia make it an attractive option for premedication. Marked side effects may include dry mouth, bradycardia and hypotension.

6.5.3 Dexmedetomidine

Dexmedetomidine is a highly selective alpha 2 receptor agonist that enhances analgesia without causing respiratory depression and generates sedation/anxiolysis, often described as being qualitatively more like a 'natural sleep' (105–108). Dosing is dictated by bioavailability and route of administration. Nasal: 1–3 mics/kg bioavailability 65%; buccal: 1–2 mics/kg bioavailability 85%; and oral: 3–5 mics/kg, a significantly higher dose reflecting a bioavailability of 16% when this route is utilised. Onset time is 25–45 minutes. It is particularly well tolerated by children as it has no taste and does not irritate mucosal membranes. Side effects include dry mouth, bradycardia and hypotension. Dexmedetomidine does not cause paradoxical agitation (109).

6.5.4 Ketamine

Ketamine achieves its clinical effect through activity at glutamate and non-NMDA receptor sites and antagonism of NMDA receptors generating sedation, dissociative anaesthesia and analgesia while preserving laryngeal reflexes, respiratory and cardiac function (110, 111). The route of administration and dose as a premed includes oral: 2–12 mg/kg; nasal: 3–5 mg/kg; IM: 5 mg/kg. Time to onset for oral administration is 20–30 minutes, nasal 10–15 minutes and IM 5–10 minutes. Oral administration of intravenous preparations of ketamine may be poorly tolerated as the solution is very bitter. Side effects include increased salivation, enhanced laryngeal reflexes, tachycardia, increased blood pressure, vivid dreams and or hallucinations.

6.5.5 Oral Morphine

Oral morphine has been used to enhance the sedative effect of other premedicants such as midazolam. However, the availability of other more effective drugs such dexmedetomidine alone or in combination with midazolam has rendered the use of morphine in this manner obsolete. Dosing for this purpose is 0.1–0.2 mg/kg. Common side effects include respiratory depression, itching, hypotension, nausea and vomiting.

6.5.6 Fentanyl

Administration of fentanyl via the oral transmucosal route, utilising a lollipop made of fentanyl mixed into a raspberry candy matrix, has been investigated as an option for anxiolytic premedication in children. Dosing for premedication is 10–20 mics/kg with an onset time of 30–45 minutes (112, 113). Side effects include nausea, vomiting and respiratory depression. As anxiolysis and increased compliance are not reliably achieved when fentanyl is deployed in this manner, it is rarely used as an anxiolytic premedicant (114).

6.5.7 Sufentanyl

Nasal sufentanyl has been studied as a potential agent for use as an anxiolytic premedicant although it is more commonly deployed in this way to provide analgesia (115). The intranasal dose is 1–2 mics/kg with an onset time of 5–10 minutes, maximal effect at 20–25 minutes and duration of 60 minutes. Sufentanyl has been utilised in combination with other agents including midazolam, ketamine and dexmedetomidine for anxiolytic premedication and for sedoanalgesia in the emergency department or dental surgery (116–118). Advantages of sufentanyl over other agents are the potency of the preparation and therefore the small volume required to deliver a therapeutic dose, its analgesic effect and the absence of taste or mucosal irritation. Side effects include nausea, vomiting and respiratory depression, particularly when administered in doses exceeding 2 mics/kg or if combined with other respiratory depressants.

Key Points

- For many children premedication represents an effective strategy for managing PIA.
- Effective anxiolytic premedication is achieved when the influence of sedation anxiolysis outweighs that of a child's anxiety.
- The dose of premedication required to successfully manage children experiencing extreme levels of anxiety may be greater than the standard published maximal dose. If these children are to be effectively premedicated, hospital protocols will need to accommodate doses above and beyond the standard maximal limit, while continuing to ensure patient safety.
- It makes little sense selecting premedication as an anxiety management strategy if the act of administering the drug generates greater anxiety than the planned intervention.
- When a combination of drugs is selected to ensure effective premedication, they should be given via a single route if at all possible. This minimises the complexity of delivery and time taken to complete the process, which in turn should minimise the risk of inflicting additional and unnecessary distress.

- Effective premedication is critically dependent upon teamwork, communication, a capacity to maintain the child's needs as the primary focus and where necessary, the ability and motivation to instantly change a plan to ensure a successful outcome.
- If premedication fails, the anxiety management strategy should be re-evaluated. The planned procedure should not simply proceed irrespective of this failure. Proceeding under such circumstances will inflict psychological trauma, damage rapport, undermine trust and may generate long-term dysfunction behaviour.
- Enforcing compliance with physical restraint when premedication fails can only be accepted as an absolute last resort when there is an inescapable valid reason that the intervention cannot be postponed and the positive benefits to the child outweigh the impact of inflicting psychological damage.
- Children with established patterns of dysfunctional behaviour following traumatic medical intervention/s will require expert elective psychological support and time to complete the therapy they will need.

Disordered Behaviour

Some disorders of behaviour can impair a child's sensitivity to, and interpretation of, others' communication and behaviour. In addition, they may fail to appreciate and observe established socially acceptable patterns of interaction, struggle to effectively explain their own thoughts and feelings and at the same time, lack the capabilities that help most of us cope with adversity.

It is worth noting that most disorders exist as a spectrum in terms of severity and many children are able to manage their anxieties with support from their family. However, some may require significant input and can suffer from levels of anxiety that are almost impossible to manage. For some, effective anxiety management strategies remain elusive.

7.1 Autistic Spectrum Disorder

Autistic spectrum disorder is defined in ICD 10 as a type of pervasive developmental disorder that is defined by the following.

1. Abnormal or impaired development that is manifest before the age of three years of age.
2. This is in addition to a characteristic type of abnormal functioning in all the three areas of psychopathology including reciprocal social interaction, communication, and restricted, stereotyped, repetitive behaviour.
3. In addition to these specific diagnostic features, a range of other nonspecific problems are common, such as phobias, sleeping and eating disturbances, temper tantrums, and (self-directed) aggression (119).

Comprehensive diagnostic criteria for autistic spectrum disorders can be found in the NICE Guideline 128, ICD 10 and DSM 5 (119–122). It is worth drawing attention to the change in classification of disorders on the autistic spectrum, adopted in DSM 5. This change brings all manifestations of autism under the same functional diagnosis of autistic spectrum disorder. As an example of the impact this has, it removes Asperger's as a separate diagnosis (123).

7.2 Stereotypical Characteristics and Anxiety Management

Characteristically there is a spectrum of impairment in communication affecting both interpretation and expression. Some children may also display impaired cognitive function and speech. Additional stereotypical characteristics may include the following.

- Avoidance of eye contact.
- Affinity for restrictive and repetitive routines and behaviour.
- An intense interest in a highly specific subject, obsessions and compulsions.

- Children who are severely affected may display maladaptive patterns of behaviour including rocking, screaming, aggression, self-harm. Manifestation of these patterns of behaviour may increase as the child becomes increasingly anxious.
- Hypersensitivity to taste is common.
- It is commonly suggested that all children with autism are hypersensitive to pain, although published literature and extensive first-hand experience does not support this.

It is important to appreciate that the level of observed impairment may increase in line with increasing anxiety. Autistic children can progress from apparently unimpaired when relaxed to completely mute, withdrawn and manifesting extreme patterns of maladaptive behaviour when extremely anxious. If changes of this nature are observed, they should be treated as an indication of increasing anxiety and an appropriate management strategy should be deployed.

It is worth noting that autism does not always exist in isolation. Autistic children may have additional diagnoses such as ADHD and or learning disabilities. This may further complicate any planned anxiety management strategy.

7.3 Attention Deficit Hyperactivity Disorder (ADHD)

Attention deficit hyperactivity disorder is defined in ICD 10 as being a hyperkinetic disorder, namely, part of a group of disorders characterized by early onset (usually in the first five years of life). There will be a lack of persistence in activities that require cognitive involvement and a tendency to move from one activity to another without completing any of them. In addition, there will be disorganised, ill-regulated, and excessive activity. Several other abnormalities may be associated. Hyperkinetic children are often reckless, impulsive, prone to accidents and find themselves in disciplinary trouble because of unthinking breaches of rules rather than deliberate defiance. Their relationships with adults are often socially disinhibited with a lack of normal caution and reserve. They may be unpopular with other children and become socially isolated. Impairment of cognitive functions is common and specific delays in motor and language development are disproportionately frequent. Secondary complications include antisocial behaviour and low self-esteem (124).

An outline of diagnostic criteria for ADHD can be found in NICE Guideline 87 published in 2018 and in ICD 10 (121, 125).

Impairment of communication in ADHD may result from inattention, an inability to concentrate and a lack of focus. Additionally, there may be extremes of behaviour due to hyperactivity and poor impulse control that will interfere with their ability to express themselves effectively.

7.4 Learning Difficulties (LD)

Learning difficulties are defined in Guideline 11 published by NICE in 2015 (126). A learning disability is defined by three core criteria:

1. Reduced intellectual ability (usually an IQ of less than 70).
2. Significant impairment of social or adaptive functioning.
3. Onset in childhood.

A child with learning difficulties may experience difficulty receiving and interpreting information, at the same time as struggling to understand and express their feelings, thoughts and experiences.

7.5 Anxiety Management Strategies

7.5.1 Management in the Community

With behaviour disorders, elective management in the community will start with evaluation of the child and include work with parents and family to increase their understanding of the condition and optimise the support they provide (126–128). An appraisal of factors in the child's environment that cause difficulty, distress or challenging behaviour will be undertaken. Following on from this, steps will be taken to minimise exposure to triggers that cause them difficulties. This involves teaching them coping strategies and helping them to develop life skills that will assist them in managing environmental stressors that cannot be removed or reduced further. Psychological support focuses on helping children develop an understanding of standard patterns of communication, to recognise their sensory deficits and utilise techniques to counterbalance them. For all children with behaviour disorders, psychological intervention is undertaken in an attempt to help the child develop greater understanding of their condition, their thoughts and emotions; their interactions with others; and to develop a greater sense of control. If anxiety and distress result in challenging behaviour, the child will be trained to deploy specific anxiety management techniques such as breathing exercises and to use their own resources such as toys, books, music and visual activity schedules to re-establish their sense of control and act as a calming influence.

7.5.2 Elective Management in Advance of Intervention

The advent of pre-assessment represents a golden opportunity to optimise the management of children with behaviour disorders.

An understanding of what care the child has received in the community and by whom is an integral part of any anxiety prevention and management strategy. Parents and carers can offer a wealth of information and add context to an understanding of a child's behaviour, needs and solutions that have been successful in the past. They will offer additional information regarding any community psychological support the child has received, resources they successfully deploy and relaxation techniques that have been established. Armed with all of this information and with the support of the parents, tailoring an appropriate and child specific anxiety management strategy for a planned medical intervention should be possible.

Consideration should be given to minimising exposure to known stressors such as prolonged starvation times, personnel invading the child's personal space, noisy or busy environments and large numbers of people. The details of any planned intervention should be shared with the child, a tailored management strategy should be agreed, and steps to ensure this strategy is followed must be taken. The ability to deploy appropriate staff and deliver timely therapeutic interventions such as play therapy and premedication, where appropriate, should be secured in advance of admission.

7.5.3 Management on the Day of Intervention

In an ideal world, as described above, a management plan should have been agreed and the resources to deliver it secured in advance. All members of the team should be aware of the intended approach. Although stereotypical patterns of communication impairment associated with each behaviour disorder are well recognised, the choice to adopt or exclude management strategies should *not* be based upon these. The approach to each and every child must be directed either by prior experience, or the dynamic, real-time appraisal of the success or failure of techniques deployed. No plan will be perfect and there is always a possibility that a plan may need to be changed on the basis of evidence and success on the day of intervention. If things are not going well, then re-evaluate and adapt accordingly.

7.5.4 Reducing Sources of Stress

Minimising fasting, delays between admission and intervention, and exposure to noisy, busy, crowded environments, while utilising known resources in the form of parents and established coping strategies, will contribute to optimal care. Choosing to schedule interventions at the beginning or end of the day, or times when plans are more likely to be successful, should be part of the management strategy. If promises are made as part of the management plan, they *must* be kept.

7.5.5 Resources

If a child has obsessions or intense interests, these may represent resources to be integrated as part of an anxiety management strategy. Engaging a child in conversation regarding their interests is likely to enhance rapport, connect with positive patterned emotional resources and act as a welcome distraction.

For some children with disordered behaviour, the use of a visual activity schedule can help reduce the distress and anxiety generated when unfamiliar or unpredictable situations are encountered (129). In children with autism, the use of these schedules may reduce the incidence of challenging behaviour (130).

7.5.6 Premedication

For children with severely disordered behaviour, premedication may be extremely effective and for some it can be the only way to manage PIA. Although benzodiazepines are routinely prescribed for children with disordered behaviour, they are known to cause paradoxical agitation in some children with autism and can cause unpredictable effects when given to children taking Ritalin or similar medication for management of ADHD. If there is concern regarding the likelihood of such a response, ketamine, clonidine and dexmedetomidine have been reported as successful alternatives. Some publications have recommended preferential use of specific agents for specific patterns of dysfunctional behaviour, yet in practice premedication of the majority of children follows standard practice by starting with midazolam and moving to alternatives if this proves less than ideal. There have been no reports of idiosyncratic responses following premedication in children with learning difficulties.

7.6 Extreme Cases

For the most severely affected children, it may be almost impossible to manage PIA. It is not uncommon to hear of children who have deteriorated from a point where they were effectively managed when attending hospital, to a situation where they refuse to leave their home and it has been established for some time that they will not accept premedication. Some may require IM ketamine sedation administered in their car outside the hospital; some may require sedation, if they will accept it, at home prior to transfer to hospital. For some, there may be no effective solution in place or imaginable. There is no magic solution for children with behaviour disorders. Each and every child is unique.

Key Points

- The majority of children with behaviour disorders will require little if any additional management beyond standard practice. Some may require time and energy intensive input. A small minority may be almost or actually impossible to manage. Irrespective of this, every child should be approached without preconceptions, treated as an individual and clinicians must display patience and compassion.
- Some behaviour disorders are characterised by an impaired communication capacity affecting both interpretation and expression.
- An observation that characteristics of a child's impairment are becoming more pronounced may indicate increasing levels of anxiety.
- Children with disordered behaviour may have anxiety management strategies that have been established to help them function in the community.
- Clinicians should specifically ask if strategies of this nature have been established as they represent a potent positive resource that may help in the management of PIA.
- Despite stereotypical characteristics associated with common syndromes, each and every one is unique. As a consequence, anxiety management strategies should be tailored to meet the needs of each individual.
- Premedication may be the best and only option to support these children, although clinicians should be aware of the potential for stereotypical idiosyncratic responses.

Family

8

Most families are a source of immense support for their children, particularly at a time of great need. As such, the family unit should be seen as a resource in the management of anxious children.

For children who have a robust, functional family unit, anxiety may be the consequence of repeated challenging and distressing experiences that they have struggled and failed to make sense of. If interventions take place when the child is very young, before they have reached a stage of cognitive development consistent with developing coping strategies, then they will struggle to integrate and cope with the experience and the consequence will be psychological trauma. This phenomenon was highlighted by Levy as far back in time as 1945. In his report, he comments on the damage done to children having surgery under the age of 3 and draws comparison between the symptoms children display and those reported by soldiers suffering from combat neurosis, known today as post-traumatic stress disorder (PTSD) (131).

In the absence of coping strategies, management of anxiety will be supportive and often requires the use of premedication each time an intervention is planned. If this approach is implemented, it may be possible to transition the child through this early vulnerable period to an age at which coping strategies can develop. In so doing, overwhelming PIA is effectively managed and associated psychological damage can be avoided.

For children without a robust or functional family unit, the likelihood they will be nurtured to develop effective coping strategies is reduced and the chances of developing dysfunctional patterns of behaviour including neuroses are increased. Under these circumstances, significant anxiety can exist in the absence of any past negative medical experiences. Naturally, the unfortunate combination of absent or dysfunctional coping strategies in addition to a history of poorly managed PIA is all too common and poses a significant challenge from an anxiety management perspective.

In the presence of significant anxieties, irrespective of the aetiology, the family unit has an important part to play in any successful management strategy. Research has demonstrated that one of the most successful interventions in the management of PIA involves pre-intervention support offering life skills coaching for child and family, delivered by an MDT (132–134).

If we accept that the family and parents have an important role to play, it is essential they understand the nature and aetiology of PIA. To achieve this, we must share the information we have gained from a century of research. In addition, we must empower parents and family by training them to function as part of the anxiety management team. It is incredible that this latter suggestion was made as long ago as 1956, by Eckenhoff when he stated:

Many doctors do not advise parents as to how best to prepare children. Adults view these matters through their own eyes, forgetting the child's outlook and making little effort at preparations.

Some parents apparently believe that the best way to handle the situation is to tell falsehoods. On a few occasions in the operating room, we have been confronted by children demanding the ice cream promised to be awaiting them.

Our experience indicates that it is important for physicians to advise parents about psychological preparation of the child. Helpful suggestions may be written with other pre-operative instructions so that parents can refer to something rather than rely on memory (17).

In recognising these considerations there is one implied adjustment we should make to current practice. In 1999 Kain alluded to this by concluding:

Anesthesiologists should make parents aware of the possibility that their child may develop negative behaviours in the 2 weeks after surgery if their child was very anxious during the induction of anesthesia (135).

In fact, by acknowledging the prevalence and consequences of PIA, we must accept it is difficult to justify failing to discuss the risk of PIA, psychological trauma and post-intervention dysfunctional behaviour as part of the consent process.

8.1 Challenging Behaviour

The child may not be the only individual who displays challenging behaviour. Parents are just as likely to require some level of management. In the first instance, it helps to recognise that the majority of such behaviour reflects the anxieties of the parent, which result as a consequence of their love and primary responsibility to protect their child. Clinicians should understand and respect this, although at times the additional burden of managing parents' behaviour can command time and resources that should be deployed in helping the child. A functional *elective* intervention strategy should help in such situations. If, despite significant supportive interventions targeting the family unit, dysfunctional and challenging behaviour persists, an adjustment to the number and identity of supporting family members may be necessary. It requires little imagination to appreciate this may be challenging to negotiate. Despite any difficulties in establishing such an adjustment, it is worth pursuing as the anxieties of a parent will contribute significantly to the anxiety of their child.

Having said all of this, it is rare that parental behaviour is so extreme that it necessitates exclusion. By offering the appropriate support, the majority of the most difficult parents or family members can evolve into a functional and positive resource that will assist in the management of their anxious child.

Key Points

- Parental anxiety stems from natural and good intentions.
- Managing parental behaviour can be resource and time intensive, but is worthwhile as it positively contributes to the management of an anxious child.
- We should inform parents of the potential psychological impact of medical interventions as the consequence of PIA.

Additional Anxiogenic Influences

The hospital environment as a whole, or aspects of it, can trigger extreme anxiety in some children, particularly following repeated exposure associated with psychological trauma. Such a process represents negative conditioning and will require expert elective psychological support if the problem is to be resolved and positive reconditioning undertaken.

For children who experience mild to moderate anxiety, there may be elements of the hospital environment and practice that have the potential, by contributing to the anxiogenic load, to push them further towards or over the threshold of a freeze–flight–fight response. Some of these elements are listed below for consideration.

As medical professionals we have, to a large extent, become desensitised to many of these aspects of care. By reconsidering these we will re-sensitise ourselves. This should empower us to consider a broader, more comprehensive range of potential negative anxiogenic stimuli when formulating anxiety management plans, which in turn should make them more effective.

9.1 Equipment

Much of the equipment we use can appear alien and frightening to a child. The literal implication of certain items such as scissors and needles may significantly contribute to anxiety at a time of maximal distress. Additionally, the proximity to items of equipment that are unfamiliar yet conform to a potentially threatening stereotype such as steel surgical instruments and anaesthetic laryngoscopes may generate additional distress. It is worth assessing the clinical environment for anything that may heighten anxiety and either remove them or hide them from view.

9.2 Clothing and Personal Protection Equipment (PPE)

Any experienced clinician will have encountered extreme negative conditioned responses to medical uniforms. Under such circumstances, the option to utilise informal attire with a view to reducing anxiety, might be considered. However, this may mean these children develop a fear of *all* individuals, as there is no longer any means to differentiate between medical professionals and everyone else.

There is some anecdotal evidence from dental practice that a general population of children, as opposed to those that are known to experience significant anxiety, may prefer some form of medical uniform to non-medical or formal attire (136–139). Additionally there may be the suggestion from such studies that the use of PPE is not a source of additional anxiety. However, it is worth noting that these studies base their comments upon questions in response to an appraisal of photographs and video rather than the results of real-time observation of clinical practice. One study that based its results on observations of clinical practice confirms a preference among children for uniforms or the use of white coats, while suggesting the use of PPE is anxiogenic (140).

There is additional evidence that a child's response to medical personal may be influenced by the colour of their uniform (141–143).

9.3 Paediatric Themes: Colour and Lighting

A great deal has been written about colour and emotion, although some of this commentary may be based on anecdotal evidence or studies with questionable research methodology (144). The behavioural response to colour may be heavily influenced by the context at the time of exposure or the result of social conditioning. Contextual influences will include how the observer feels, the situation they are in or even if it's day or night. An example of social conditioning would be our response to the colour red which is stereotypically used to indicate a warning or to tell us to 'STOP'. Published commentary on this subject repeatedly references the colour red making us more alert and the colour black being linked to fear, death or something sinister. Interestingly, as black becomes a colour regularly deployed as being cool or efficient and linked to martial arts, there appears to be a gender response, seen more commonly in boys, towards perceiving this colour in a positive light (145). Other examples of commonly encountered themes in research include the positive appraisal of the colour yellow by both sexes, the perception of the colour blue as soothing and calming, that a shade of pink known as Baker–Miller pink suppresses aggression and that the saturation of colour or vibrancy is associated with arousal (146–148).

How we utilise this information continues to be a subject of considerable debate. There is enough evidence to suggest that we might avoid bright vibrant colours, avoid using red or black, and seek to utilise soothing shades of pastel yellow, blue or Baker–Miller pink in areas where children are likely to experience PIA. However, this would run counter to common opinion that the décor in all clinical paediatric areas should be bright and colourful, with plenty of illustrations depicting popular characters from books, games, films and television. Perhaps a pragmatic solution is to utilise bright and colourful decoration for most 'general' clinical areas, and subtle, less vibrant pastel shades of soft neutral colour in areas where children are expected to rest, recover, or undergo medical interventions.

Lighting levels in the clinical environment are an additional influence with regards to the effective management of PIA. Fear of the dark and an understanding of the sensory consequences of low lighting levels are such that we can all appreciate that a darkened environment may appear threatening to an anxious child. On the other hand, reducing light intensity may be helpful if we are seeking to calm an anxious child after any perceived threat has passed. Other situations where a darkened room may assist in supporting a child include during the onset or recovery phase of sedation, and when a child is trying to rest or sleep.

9.4 Other Children and Procedures: Sight and Sound

As we know, anxiety heightens the senses. An anxious child will experience a heightened sensitivity to what they see and hear. In addition, they will tend to interpret these as an indication of potential threat until they know, unequivocally, that they are safe. If an anxious child observes or hears another child in distress, they may assume they will have a similar experience with a similar outcome. Additionally, they are unlikely to enjoy observing or listening to medical interventions that are taking place. With this in mind, we should carefully consider and plan the workflow and patient journey through clinical areas to minimise ambient noise and avoid children seeing or hearing other patients undergoing or recovering from medical interventions. When seeking to optimise a clinical space, particularly those used for transit and recovery after medical interventions, it is worth considering the use of positive auditory stimuli, including music therapy or ambient sound that has stereotypical positive associations, with a view to exerting a positive subliminal influence upon mood.

9.5 Taste and Odour

As described with regards to premedication, some medications are less than palatable. Additionally, many drugs have a distinctive if not unpleasant smell. These sensory stimuli may represent an additional negative stimulus for anxious children or become a distinctive focal point associated with a negative conditioned behavioural response. The smell of the hospital environment itself can similarly become associated with repetitive negative experiences. Consideration should be given to such influences when seeking to implement anxiety management strategies.

9.6 Temperature and Tactile Stimuli

The ambient temperature and general physical comfort of the environment will have some effect upon children with heightened sensitivity. In isolation, their contribution to outcome will be slight, yet they may exert an additional positive or negative influence upon outcome.

Key Points

- Hospital equipment may frighten children. We should evaluate our working area for anything that might generate additional and unwanted distress. Where possible these should be removed or obscured.
- There is incomplete evidence suggesting children prefer clinicians to wear some form of uniform.
- Items of PPE may cause additional distress.
- Anxiety heightens all of the senses. What children see, hear, smell, taste and feel can have a significant negative influence upon them if we fail to manage these aspects of a child's environment effectively.
- It may be possible to optimise visual and auditory stimuli in the form of colour and sound to exert positive subliminal influence and generate a sense of calm.

Chapter 1

Elective Management

Optimum care for anxious children mandates deployment of anxiety management strategies *in advance* of planned interventions. For this to be achieved, we must detect children who are more likely to experience anxiety by utilising an effective screening system. The advent of pre-assessment grants the perfect opportunity to implement such a system with a view to offering specialist psychological support and intervention to those who need it.

Generally, the majority of children entering a hospital environment will experience mild to moderate anxiety, which could be described as a 'normal', appropriate and understandable level of apprehension under the circumstances. Most of these children can be managed with standard or minimally augmented supportive measures such as extra time and effort to ensure rapport and trust have been established, or the deployment of premedication. A smaller proportion of children, with significant anxieties and or established patterns of dysfunctional behaviour, are likely to require expert, complex and time-consuming psychological support from specialist services which, in most institutions, are already working at or beyond their maximum capacity. With all things considered, if we are to effectively manage anxious children while ensuring efficient and appropriate use of finite resources, it cannot fall to specialist services to manage patient screening and triage. The solution is to integrate these processes into the standard patient pathway. This will ensure specialist services only receive referrals for those needing more intensive input, while all other children are highlighted for management by the regular team.

After considering these aspects of anxiety management, an optimum patient pathway may require the following:

- All clinicians to maintain a core competency in the management of mild and moderate anxiety.
- A screening system to highlight children who, as the consequence of extreme anxiety or established patterns of dysfunctional behaviour, require specialist psychological support.
- An ability to triage cases to ensure only those who really need specialist psychological support are referred for assessment and intervention.
- A capacity for real-time coordination and adjustment of standard or augmented management strategies.
- Post-discharge follow-up to highlight children who have sustained psychological trauma necessitating further intervention.

Naturally, optimising the patient pathway may require deployment of additional resources, time and money. However, as a preventive initiative, such investment should reduce morbidity and long-term costs through improvements in quality and efficiency of care.

10.1 Anxiety Management Services

Anxiety management services exist in some form in most paediatric units although the extent and structure varies significantly. Few, if any units have the luxury of a fully funded and recognised multidisciplinary team (MDT) with established patient pathways. Most units have a loose conglomerate of specialists who work as a dispersed MDT, communicating and coordinating care on a case-by-case basis yet still managing to deliver effective support and improved outcomes. Some units have few or no resources, no play specialists and extremely limited access to specialist psychological support. Internationally, the focus for clinical intervention also varies considerably between input purely from psychological services, to units where input takes the form of anaesthetic-led hypnotherapy.

When one considers the prevalence of PIA, the associated morbidity, evidence that there are interventions we can make to reduce this morbidity, and finally our duty of care to children who have already sustained emotional trauma following medical intervention, is it not time we sought uniformity and quality in the management of anxious children? To achieve such a goal, we must define standards of practice, reach consensus regarding the anatomy of anxiety management services and commit resources to deliver optimum care. With regards to the anatomy of anxiety management services, at very least one might argue there should be representation from the departments of psychology, possibly psychiatry, play therapy, anaesthesia and nursing. Additionally, the capacity to service research and audit will be essential in time.

10.2 Elective Therapy

Naturally, all elective interventions are aimed at reducing anxiety. Bearing in mind every child is unique and that the aetiology of anxiety will vary from one child to the next, elective intervention and support strategies will encompass a myriad of techniques. Where possible and appropriate, interventions will seek to target an underlying cause for enhanced anxiety. Elective interventions may utilise the following.

- Time to build rapport and trust away from anxiogenic stimuli.
- Time to establish a clear understanding of all issues including those that relate to the family unit as a whole and the full extended history of anxiety.
- Behaviour modification through reconditioning and relearning.
- Real or projected graduated exposure therapy for extreme phobic responses.
- Behaviour modification by challenging and readjusting a child's understanding and perception of an anxiogenic stimulus.
- In the absence of effective coping strategies, work to develop existing or new strategies utilising existing positive resources if they exist.
- Training in the management of the physical manifestations of anxiety such as relaxation and breathing techniques may be offered as part of any supportive intervention.

Interventions should nurture *independent* coping strategies where possible. Replacing one vulnerability with another, in the form of dependence upon individuals or a restrictive and ritualistic process, does not address the underlying issue unless it is a support structure for relearning that will empower the child.

It is worth appreciating that PIA, particularly in those most severely affected, may be a specific or primary manifestation of a global malignant anxiety disorder, one that is at first triggered in a specific area of the child's life. It then evolves to invade, impair and disable multiple or all areas of a child's life. Any attempted therapeutic intervention that fails to address the underlying issue, cause and process in such children is likely to fail in the longer term. From a quality of life perspective, these children need our help. Our goal is not simply to complete a desired medical intervention, then move on. It is to manage and care for the child holistically, in mind and body. When this is achieved, such children flourish, grow and develop an independent constitutional resilience that is formidable. With time, this capacity empowers them to reclaim and repair all aspects of their lives that were crippled before. If they achieve this, they will often go on to evolve as individuals in a manner that would have been inconceivable prior to this transformation.

10.3 Therapeutic Interventions

10.3.1 Psychology

Psychological input and support forms the backbone of most if not all elective psychological intervention currently on offer. The option to seek support from a dedicated and appropriately funded psychology service is essential when seeking to manage an anxious child.

Techniques that are commonly deployed in the management of anxiety include (149) the following.

- **Cognitive Behaviour Therapy (CBT)** – How we think about things affects how we feel, behave and communicate. CBT seeks to address negative ideation by encouraging positive thought and perspective, by helping children to develop coping strategies, with a view to nurturing positive functional feelings, behaviour and communication.
- **Psychodynamic and Psychoanalytic Therapy** – Seeks to pinpoint, understand and dismantle defence mechanisms and negative behaviour that has evolved as a consequence of past experiences and relationships.
- **Humanistic and Grief Therapy, Transactional Analysis (TA)** (150, 151) – Based upon the theory that individuals have control over their own reality and actions, they offer a framework for understanding established patterns of behaviour and a means to implement new ones.
- **Interpersonal (Integrative) Therapy** – Analysis and understanding of interpersonal relationships and communication to minimise conflict and patterns of dysfunctional behaviour.
- **Family Therapy** – On its own or in addition to other interventions. It targets the family unit with a view to minimising negative and maximising positive influence and support.

If anxiety manifests as a phobic response, typical interventions will include:

- **CBT**
- **Exposure Desensitisation** – Imagined or in real-life.
- **Modelling behaviour** – Watching recordings or real-life examples of individuals coping with exposure to the phobic stimulus.

Psychological support may also employ other therapies including Neurolinguistic Programming (NLP) (152–154) and hypnotherapy.

10.3.2 Play Specialists

Play specialists are an invaluable and vital part of the MDT. They are almost certainly *the* only medical professionals whose sole role is to interact 24/7 with the child, with a view to ensuring their psychological and emotional wellbeing. They do this through engagement in play and other supportive activities. They devote an immense amount of time towards connecting with the child and family, building rapport and establishing an understanding of their history, thoughts, feeling and needs.

As a consequence, play specialists represent an invaluable resource offering a wealth of information that significantly contributes to the management of anxious children. Their position is unique in light of their capacity to act as a bridge between child, family and the clinical team. Their input and recommendations should always be respected and considered when formulating an anxiety management strategy. Their inclusion within any anxiety management service should be compulsory.

10.3.3 Play Therapists

Play therapists offer therapeutic intervention on an elective basis in a similar manner to psychologists. They offer therapy through play, helping children appraise and understand their feelings and thoughts with a view to nurturing positive thinking, feelings, behaviour and independent coping strategies (155).

10.3.4 Hypnotherapy

Hypnotherapy utilises an altered state of consciousness, characterised by trance logic, where thoughts and concepts are appraised literally, whilst conscious critical appraisal is suspended. This enhances the potency of therapeutic interventions. Interventions deployed include those from other frameworks of practice such as CBT, NLP, TA, exposure desensitisation, guided imagery, modelling behaviour through storytelling and imagination, psychodynamic therapy and psychoanalysis, in addition to techniques specific to hypnotherapy including regression, dissociation and pseudo-orientation.

Trance phenomena grant the additional advantages of accelerating relearning, accelerating and enhancing acceptance of alternate perspectives and the potential for change. Therapy characteristically includes ego boosting and the installation of post-hypnotic suggestions that are consistent with the desired therapeutic outcome.

Lastly, it is worth noting that research suggests hypnotherapy has a significant positive effect on recovery following surgery and is more effective than midazolam with regards to reducing anxiety at induction of anaesthesia and signs of emotional trauma following surgery (93, 156, 157).

10.4 Preparation Programmes

The goal of preparation programmes is to pre-empt and manage regular anxiety generated by the unfamiliar and unexpected, in addition to offering therapeutic support and intervention for more complex patients. Although patient satisfaction is an inevitable and welcome consequence of any additional supportive input, it is not in itself an indication of reduced anxiety and consequent psychological trauma.

Preparation programmes must offer evidence-based, cost and resource efficient interventions, that reduce anxiety and psychological trauma for all children. If we are to achieve this, we must recognise that the nature and intensity of interventions required to manage mild or moderate anxiety differ significantly from those required to manage extreme anxiety of complex aetiology. As such, any successful, clinically effective and resource efficient preparation programme must deliver generic care for the majority while ensuring appropriate and intensive interventions are offered to those with more complex needs.

10.5 Commonly Deployed Interventions

Interventions commonly deployed, in order of *decreasing* efficacy include life or coping skills training, modelling or shaping, play therapy, hospital tours and lastly printed materials (158, 159). Additionally, video recordings have been used to deliver many of these strategies.

10.5.1 Life and Coping Skills Training

Perhaps the most commonly cited and successful preparation programmes utilise life skills training to nurture coping strategies in the child and the family unit. Training may be intensive and specifically tailored to address underlying psychological issues which will likely suit children experiencing severe anxiety with an underlying cause. However, offering such intervention to all children is likely unnecessary and inefficient with regards use of valuable finite resources. With this in mind, some programmes, such as Kain's ADVANCE programme, are designed to deliver psychological interventions of known efficacy, to all children and families while minimising cost, hospital attendance and demand upon finite resources. The aim of the programme was to reduce anxiety, use video to educate and model behaviour, offer exposure/shaping therapy, encourage parental presence at induction of anaesthesia, coach parents in distraction and the avoidance of excessive reassurance, while training them to nurture life skills and coping strategies. Following this intervention, there was a statistically significant reduction in anxiety and improved outcome (160).

We should note that Kaine's research suggests that history of medical intervention, timing of delivery in relation to the planned procedure and the age of the recipient, significantly influences programme efficacy (161). Preparation may *increase* anxiety for children under the age of 3 years and those with a history of hospital admission or prior medical intervention. Additionally, children over 6 years of age should receive preparation a week or more in advance of planned procedures.

Finally, we should recognise there is a great deal of research and work to be done with regards to establishing, agreeing and implementing optimal frameworks for practice. As hospital care is streamlined and children travel further to access centralised specialist care, the use of technology and novel media to deploy interventions of proven efficacy will evolve (162).

10.5.2 Hospital Tours and Written Information

Despite being one of the least effective interventions, hospital tours and written information are used in many institutions as they are cheap and can be delivered by staff with little or no psychological training. In mitigation, there is nothing to prevent any opportunity for patient interaction from being used to deliver conversational or formal therapy by staff with appropriate skills. Additionally, hospital tours and written material may reduce anxiety by educating, familiarising and therefore desensitising the child and family with regards to an unfamiliar hospital environment, staff and procedures. Naturally, such benefits can only be realised if there is full engagement with the planned intervention.

Lastly, we must appreciate children have an infinite capacity for dissociation and fantasy. As such, it is possible for a child to read material or visit hospital, yet consciously or unconsciously avoid processing and associating such interventions with forthcoming procedures.

10.5.3 Audio Visual

Video and auditory material can be used to deliver anything from carefully designed complex psychological interventions to basic information. Content that offers actual footage of the hospital the child will be attending, with actors successfully and calmly negotiating the intended process (offering modelling behaviour), are more effective than generic content, in terms of reducing anxiety and post-hospital dysfunctional behaviour (163–166).

Audio material can deliver anything from basic information to specialist therapeutic content in the form of spoken therapy. For maximal effect, therapeutic material should be used repeatedly and at a time when it will command the recipient's full attention, such as last thing at night while drifting off to sleep. For maximal effect, content should bespoke, meet the needs of the individual, utilise any positive resources they already have and nurture those they need and are yet to develop.

10.6 Evolving Technology

10.6.1 Virtual and Augmented Reality

Virtual reality (VR) can be deployed for simple distraction or as part of a carefully designed preparation programme offering modelling, exposure and desensitisation. Although studies have been small, of varied quality and methodology, results suggest VR can reduce pain and anxiety when used to prepare for, or distract during procedures (167).

The influence of VR lies in its capacity to generate an 'immersive' environment that appears so realistic, we interact and behave as we would in real life. As a consequence, VR represents a potent tool for the management of phobia through exposure desensitisation and for use in remodelling behaviour.

Augmented reality (AR) offers a means to project virtual elements upon real surroundings. Examples might include imaginary friends that follow and support children throughout hospital activity or the projection of superheroes that replace members of staff (168). We should note, the influence of AR relates to distraction and an ability to superimpose the novel or familiar upon unfamiliar surroundings. AR does not generate an immersive experience.

10.6.2 Apps

Once developed, apps offer a means to ensure maximal access to anxiety management strategies, while minimising cost and the need for specialist input (169, 170). It is important to appreciate, as for all media, the value of the medium or conduit lies in its capacity to optimise delivery of the therapeutic content. It is then the content that ultimately dictates efficacy. As such, apps that are carefully constructed tools for the purposes of delivering psychological interventions of known efficacy will offer greater benefit than those that simply deliver generic information.

To date, although research examining the benefits of apps in the management of PIA is in its infancy, results so far suggest further investigation is warranted (163, 171, 172).

Key Points

- Elective preparation is preventive and should be utilised as a foundation in the management of PIA.
- The most effective way to reduce PIA and consequent psychological trauma is to deploy interventions that dismantle underlying dysfunctional processes and nurture life skills or coping strategies.
- Children with complex causes for more extreme anxiety will almost certainly require more intensive and time-consuming interventions from specialist clinicians.
- Delivering complex interventions to all children is unnecessary and, for some children, would represent an inappropriate use of finite, valuable resources.
- A system of triage will be required to ensure all children receive the level of input they require while ensuring the efficient use of resources.
- Nature and content of interventions rather than the medium dictate efficacy.
- Most if not all research projects have studied the impact of interventions in a mixed general population. As a consequence, we must be cautious when applying recommendations from such research in small subpopulations, such as children with extreme anxiety of complex aetiology.
- Research comparing the efficacy of different intervention strategies is incomplete.
- The success and efficacy of any intervention will be critically dependent upon child and family engagement.

References

1. Spielberger CD. *State-Trait Anxiety Inventory for Children: Preliminary Manual.* (Palo Alto, CA: Consulting Psychologists Press, 1973).

2. Rigoli F, Ewbank M, Dalgleish T and Calder A. Threat visibility modulates the defensive brain circuit underlying fear and anxiety. *Neurosci Lett.* [Internet]. 2016;612:7–13. Available from http://dx.doi.org/10.1016/j.neulet.2015.11.026.

3. Navarro J and Marvin K. *What Every BODY Is Saying: An Ex-FBI Agent's Guide to Speed Reading People.* [Internet]. (New York: Harper Collins, 2008, pp. 27–34). Available from www.harpercollins.ca/9780061438295/what-every-body-is-saying.

4. Faber ESL, Delaney AJ, Power JM, Sedlak PL, Crane JW and Sah P. Modulation of SK channel trafficking by beta adrenoceptors enhances excitatory synaptic transmission and plasticity in the amygdala. *J Neurosci.* 2008;22;28(43):10803–13.

5. McIntyre CK and Roozendaal B. Adrenal stress hormones and enhanced memory for emotionally arousing experiences. In: *Neural Plasticity and Memory: From Genes to Brain Imaging.* [Internet]. (Boca Raton, FL: CRC Press/Taylor & Francis, 2007, pp. 17–19). Available from www.ncbi.nlm.nih.gov/pubmed/21204426.

6. McGaugh JL, Cahill L and Roozendaal B. Involvement of the amygdala in memory storage: interaction with other brain systems. *Proc Natl Acad Sci.* 2002;93(24):13508–14.

7. Rudolph KD, Dennig MD and Weisz JR. Determinants and consequences of children's coping in the medical setting: conceptualization, review, and critique. *Psychol Bull.* 1995;118(3):328–57.

8. Tulving E. Episodic memory: from mind to brain. *Annu Rev Psychol.* [Internet]. 2002 Feb 1;53(1):1–25. Available from https://doi.org/10.1146/annurev.psych.53.100901.135114.

9. Dickerson BC and Eichenbaum H. The episodic memory system: neurocircuitry and disorders. *Neuropsychopharmacology.* 2010;35(1):86–104.

10. Wright KD, Stewart SH, Finley GA and Buffett-Jerrott SE. Prevention and intervention preoperative anxiety in children: a critical review. *Behav Modif.* 2007;31(1):52–79.

11. Kain ZN, Wang SM, Hofstadter MB, Mayes LC and Caramico LA. Distress during the induction of anesthesia and postoperative behavioral outcomes. *Anesth Analg.* 1999;88:1042–7.

12. Uki K and Daaboul DG. Postoperative maladaptive behavioral changes in children. *Middle East J Anaesthesiol.* 2011;21(2):183–92.

13. Kotiniemi LH, Ryhänen PT and Moilanen IK. Behavioural changes in children following day-case surgery: a 4-week follow-up of 551 children. *Anaesthesia.* 1997;52(10):970–6.

14. Karling M, Stenlund H and Hagglof B. Child behaviour after anaesthesia: associated risk factors. *Acta Paediatr.* [Internet]. 2007;96(5):740–7. Available from www.ncbi.nlm.nih.gov/pubmed/17462064.

15. Kain ZN, Mayes LC, O'Connor TZ and Cicchetti DV. Preoperative anxiety in children: predictors and outcomes. *JAMA Pediatr.* [Internet]. 1996 Dec 1;150(12):1238–45. Available from https://doi.org/10.1001/archpedi.1996.02170370016002.

16. Levy DM. Psychic trauma of operations in children. *JAMA Pediatr.* [Internet]. 1945;69(1):7–25. Available from https://jamanetwork.com/journals/jamapediatrics/article-abstract/1180027.

17. Eckenhoff JE. Relationship of anesthesia to postoperative personality changes in children. *AMA Am J Dis Child.* [Internet]. 1953;86(5):587–91. Available from https://jamanetwork.com/journals/

jamapediatrics/article-abstract/496484? resultClick=1.

18. Vernon DTA, Schulman JL and Foley JM. Changes in children's behavior after hospitalization: some dimensions of response and their correlates. *Am J Dis Child.* 1966;111(6): 581–93.

19. Stipic SS, Carev M, Kardum G, Roje Z, Litre DM and Elezovic N. Are postoperative behavioural changes after adenotonsillectomy in children influenced by the type of anaesthesia? *Eur J Anaesthesiol.* 2015;32(5):311–19.

20. Lewis SJ, Arseneault L, Caspi A, et al. The epidemiology of trauma and post-traumatic stress disorder in a representative cohort of young people in England and Wales. *The Lancet Psychiatry* [Internet]. 2019;6(3):247–56. Available from http://dx .doi.org/10.1016/S2215–0366(19)30031-8.

21. Frissa S, Hatch SL, Gazard B and Hotopf M. Trauma and current symptoms of PTSD in a South East London community. *Soc Psychiatr Psychiatric Epidemiol.* 2013; DOI: 10.1007/s001127-013-0689-8.

22. Felitti VJ, Anda RF, Nordenberg D, et al. Relationship of childhood abuse and household dysfunction to many of the leading causes of death in adults: the Adverse Childhood Experiences (ACE) Study. *Am J Prev Med.* [Internet]. 1998 May 1;14(4):245–58. Available from https://doi.org/10.1016/S0749–3797(98) 00017-8.

23. Colich NL, Rosen ML, Williams ES and McLaughlin KA. Biological aging in childhood and adolescence following experiences of threat and deprivation: a systematic review and meta-analysis. *Psychol Bull.* 2020;146(9):721–64.

24. ONS. UK Population. *Soc Trends.* [Internet]. 2011;41(1):1–19. Available from www.palgrave-journals.com/doifinder/10 .1057/st.2011.2.

25. Hunt SD and Nevin JR. Power in a channel of distribution: sources and consequences. *J Mark Res.* 2006;11(2):186.

26. Katsakou C. Coercion and treatment satisfaction among involuntary patients. *APA* 2010;61(3). Published Online:1 Mar

2010. https://doi.org/10.1176/ps.2010.61.3 .286.

27. Mohr WK, Petti TA and Mohr BD. Adverse effects associated with physical restraint. *Can J Psychiatr.* [Internet]. 2003;48(5):330–7. Available from www .embase.com/search/results?subaction= viewrecord&from=export&id=L36841271.

28. Tan L and Meakin GH. Anaesthesia for the uncooperative child. *Contin Educ Anaesthesia Crit Care Pain.* 2010;10(2): 48–52.

29. Royal College of Nursing. *Let's Talk about Restraint.* (London: RCN, 2008).

30. Birdwhistell RL. *Introduction to Kinesics: An Annotation System for Analysis of Body Motion and Gesture.* (Louisville, KY: University of Louisville, 1952).

31. Hall ET. The anthropology of space: an organizing model. In: *The Hidden Dimension.* (New York: Doubleday, 1966, pp. 108–9).

32. Fast J. How we handle space. In: *Body Language: How Our Movements and Posture Reveal Our Inner Secret Selves.* (Lanham, MD: M. Evans & Company, 2002).

33. Mehrabian A. Significance of posture and position in the communication of attitude and status relationships. *Psychol Bull.* 1969;71(5):359–72.

34. Burgoon JK and Carroll CE. Expectancy violations theory. In: *The International Encyclopedia of Interpersonal Communication.* (Hoboken, NJ: John Wiley, 2015, p. 9). Available from https:// doi.org/10.1002/9781118540190.wbeic102.

35. Fast J. Of animals and territory. In: *Body Language: How Our Movements and Posture Reveal Our Inner Secret Selves.* (Lanham, MD: M. Evans & Company, 2002, pp. 9–18).

36. Argyle M and Dean J. Eye contact, distance and affiliation. *Sociometry.* 1965;28 (3):289–304.

37. Fast J. Winking, blinking and nods. In: *Body Language: How Our Movements and Posture Reveal Our Inner Secret Selves.* (M. Evans & Company, 2002, pp. 9–19).

38. Goffman E. Facial engagements. In: Mortensen D, ed., *Communication Theory*. (Routledge, 2017, 27 pp.)

39. Burgoon JK, Manusov V, Mineo P and Hale JL. Effects of gaze on hiring, credibility, attraction and relational message interpretation. *J Nonverbal Behav*. 1985;9(3):133–46.

40. Chris S. The effects of nonverbal behavior on outcomes of compliance gaining attempts. *Commun Stud*. 1993;44(3–4): 169–87.

41. Ekman P. Universals and cultural differences in facial expressions of emotion. In: Cole J, ed., *Nebraska Symposium on Motivation*. [Internet]. (Lincoln: University of Nebraska Press, 1972, pp. 207–82). Available from www.paulekman.com.

42. Ekman P. Universal facial expressions of emotion. *Calif Ment Heal Res Dig*. [Internet]. 1970;4(8):151–8. Available from www.paulekman.com/resources/journal-articles.

43. Scheflen A. The significance of posture in communication systems. In: Mortensen CD, ed., *Communication Theory*. (Routledge, 2008, 13 pp.)

44. Harrigan JA and Rosenthal R. Physicians' head and body positions as determinants of perceived rapport. *J Appl Soc Psychol*. 1983;13(6):496–509.

45. Mehrabian A. Communicating without words. In: Mortensen CD, ed., *Communication Theory*. (Routledge, 2008, 8 pp.)

46. Eerland A, Guadalupe TM, Franken IHA and Zwaan RA. Posture as index for approach-avoidance behavior. *PLoS ONE*. 2012;7(2):1–5.

47. Beck RS, Daughtridge R and Sloane PD. Physician–patient communication in the primary care office. A systematic Review. *J Am Board Family Pract*. 15(1):25–38.

48. Scheflin A. The significance of posture in communication systems. In: Mortensen CD, ed., *Communication Theory*. (Routledge, 2008), 13 pp.

49. Sommer R. Studies in personal space. *Sociometry*. [Internet]. 1959;22(3):247–60.

Available from www.jstor.org/stable/2785668.

50. Robinson J. Getting down to business talk, gaze, and body orientation during openings of doctor–patient consultations. *Hum Commun Res*. 1998;25(1):97–123.

51. Robinson JD. Nonverbal communication and physician–patient interaction. In: *The Sage Handbook of Non-Verbal Communication*. (Sage Publications, 2006, pp. 437–59).

52. Fast J. An alphabet for movement. In: *Body Language: How Our Movements and Posture Reveal Our Inner Secret Selves*. (Pocket Books, 2003, p. 148).

53. Barbosa CD, Balp MM, Kulich K, Germain N and Rofail D. A literature review to explore the link between treatment satisfaction and adherence, compliance, and persistence. *Patient Prefer Adherence*. 2012;6:39–48.

54. Burgoon JK, Pfau M, Parrott R, Birk T, Coker R and Burgoon M. Relational communication, satisfaction, compliance-gaining strategies, and compliance in communication between physicians and patients. *Commun Monogr*. 1987;54(3): 307–24.

55. Burgoon JK and Bacue A. Nonverbal communication skills. In: Greene JO and Burleson BR, eds., *Handbook of Communication and Social Interaction Skills*. (Routledge, 2003).

56. Sikorski W. Paralinguistic communication in the therapeutic relationship. *Arch Psychiatry Psychother*. 2012;14(1):49–54.

57. Knowlton GE and Larkin KT. The influence of voice volume, pitch, and speech rate on progressive relaxation training: application of methods from speech pathology and audiology. *Appl Psychophysiol Biofeedback*. 2006;31(2): 173–85.

58. Remacle A, Todovora T and Zambra N. The acoustic correlates of hypnotic voice. In: 12th Pan European Voice Conference. [Internet] 2017. Available from http://hdl .handle.net/2268/214666.

59. Boag S. Conscious, preconscious, and unconscious. In: Zeigler-Hill V and

Shackelford TK, eds., *Encyclopedia of Personality and Individual Differences.* (Springer, 2017, pp. 1–8).

60. Erickson M and Rossi E. Two level communication and the microdynamics of trance and suggestion. *Am J Clin Hypnosis.* 1976;18(3):153–71.

61. Erickson MH and Rossi EL. The indirect forms of suggestion. In: *Hypnotherapy an Exploratory Casebook.* (John Wiley, 1979, pp. 30–58).

62. Simpkins C and Simpkins AM. An exploratory outcome comparison between an Ericksonian approach to therapy and brief dynamic therapy. *Am J Clin Hypn.* 2008;50(3):217–32.

63. *The Collected Works of Milton H. Erickson* [Internet]. Available from https://catalog .erickson-foundation.org/page/collected-works-2605.

64. Short D. Conversational hypnosis: conceptual and technical differences relative to traditional hypnosis. *Am J Clin Hypn.* 2018;61(2):125–39.

65. Cambridge English Dictionary. [Internet]. Cambridge University Press. Available from https://dictionary.cambridge.org/ dictionary/english/implication.

66. Merriam-Webster Dictionary Implication. [Internet]. Available from www.merriam-webster.com/dictionary/implication.

67. Erickson MH and Rossi EL. The utilization approach: Trance induction and suggestion. In: *Hypnotherapy: An Exploratory Casebook.* (John Wiley, 1979, pp. 59–85).

68. Rossi EL. Further clinical techniques of hypnosis: utilization techniques. In: *The Collected Papers of Milton H. Erickson, Volume 1.* (Milton H. Erikson Foundation Press, 1980, pp. 177–205).

69. Cyna AM, Andrew MI and Tan SGM. Communication skills for the anaesthetist. *Anaesthesia.* 2009;64(6): 658–65.

70. Newton DA, Walther J and Jamesbaesler E. Nonverbal expectancy violations and conversational involvement. *J Nonverbal Behav.* 1989;13:97–119.

71. Burgoon JK, Dunbar NE and Segrin C. Nonverbal influence. In: Dillard JP and Pfau M, eds., *The Persuasion Handbook: Developments in Theory and Practice.* (Thousand Oaks, CA: Sage, 2002, pp. 445–74).

72. Patterson M., Powell JU and Lenihan MG. Touch, compliance, and interpersonal affect. *J Nonverbal Behav.* 1986;10(1): 41–50.

73. Guéguen N. Status, apparel and touch: Their joint effects on compliance to a request. *North Am J Psychol.* 2002;4:279–86.

74. Goldman M, Kiyohara O and Pfannensteil D. Interpersonal touch, social labeling and foot-in-the-door effect. *J Soc Psychol.* 125(2):143–7.

75. Erickson MH and Rossi EL. The confusion-restructuring approach. In: *Hypnotic Realities The Induction of Clinical Hypnosis and Forms of Indirect Suggestion.* (New York: Irvington Publishers, 1976, pp. 115–16).

76. Yapko MD. Induction through confusion techniques. In: *Trancework: An Introduction to the Practice of Clinical Hypnosis*, 4th ed. (Routledge, 2012, pp. 324–8).

77. Erickson M, Rossi EL and Rossi SI. *Hypnotic Realities: The Induction of Clinical Hypnosis and Forms of Indirect Suggestion.* [Internet]. (Irvington Publishers,1976). Available from www .amazon.co.uk/Hypnotic-Realities-Induction-Clinical-Suggestion.

78. Erickson MH and Rossi EL. *Hypnotherapy: An Exploratory Casebook.* [Internet]. (John Wiley & Sons, 1979). Available from www .amazon.co.uk/Hypnotherapy-Exploratory-Casebook-Milton-Erickson/dp/ 0470265957.

79. Yapko MD. *Trancework: An Introduction to the Practice of Clinical Hypnosis*, 4th ed. (Routledge, 2012).

80. Erickson MH. Pseudo-orientation in time as an hypnotherapeutic procedure. *J Clin Exp Hypn.* [Internet]. 1954 Oct 1;2(4): 261–83. Available from https://doi.org/10 .1080/00207145408410117.

81. Hall KD and Cook MH. The Power of Validation: Arming Your Child against Bullying, Peer Pressure, Addiction, Self-Harm and Out-of-Control Emotions. 2012. Epub ISBN 9781608826254. Available from Kindle Books.

82. Linehan MM. Validation and psychotherapy. Empathy reconsidered. *New Dir Psychother.* [Internet]. 1997;353–92. Available from http://content.apa.org/books/10226-016.

83. Carette S, Fiola JL, Charest M-C, et al. Guided imagery for adolescent post-spinal fusion pain management: A pilot study. *Pain Manag Nurs.* [Internet]. 2015;16(3): 211–20. Available from http://onlinelibrary.wiley.com/o/cochrane/clcentral/articles/503/CN-01367503/frame.html.

84. Felix MM. dos S, Ferreira MBG, Oliveira LF de, Barichello E, Pires P da S and Barbosa MH. Guided imagery relaxation therapy on preoperative anxiety: a randomized clinical trial. *Rev Lat Am Enfermagem.* 2018;26.

85. Stanley JM, Galloway JP, Clair AA and Jellison J. The effects of music assisted relaxation on preoperative anxiety. *J Music Ther.* 1995;XXXII(1):2–21.

86. Vagnoli L, Bettini A, Amore E, De Masi S and Messeri A. Relaxation-guided imagery reduces perioperative anxiety and pain in children: a randomized study. *Eur J Pediatr.* 2019;168(2)186–9.

87. Statement of 1892 by a Committee appointed by the Council of the BMA. *Suppl to BMJ.* 1955;Appendix X:190–3.

88. Medical Use of Hypnotism: Report of a Subcommittee appointed by the Psychological Medicine Group Committee of the British Medical Association. *Suppl to BMJ.* 1955;Appendix X:190–3.

89. Council on Mental Health: Medical use of hypnosis. *JAMA.* 1958;168(2):186–9.

90. Jiang H, White MP, Greicius MD, Waelde LC and Spiegel D. Brain activity and functional connectivity associated with hypnosis. *Cereb Cortex.* 2017;27(8): 4083–93.

91. Practice C and Rogovik AL. Pediatric pearls hypnosis for treatment of pain in children. *Can Fam Physician.* [Internet]. 2007;53(5): 823–5. Available from www.pubmedcentral.nih.gov/articlerender.fcgi?artid=1949166&tool=pmcentrez&rendertype=abstract.

92. Birnie KA, Ons BAH, Noel M, et al. Systematic review and meta-analysis of distraction and hypnosis for needle-related pain and distress in children and adolescents. *J Pediatr Psychol.* 2014;39(8): 783–808.

93. Schnur JB, Kafer I, Marcus C and Montgomery GH. Hypnosis to manage distress related to medical procedures: a meta-analysis. *NCBI.* 2009;25:114–28.

94. Butler LD, Symons BK, Henderson SL, Shortliffe LD and Spiegel D. Hypnosis reduces distress and duration of an invasive medical procedure for children. *Pediatrics.* 2017;115(1):e77–85.

95. Montgomery GH, Duhamel KN and Redd WH. A meta-analysis of hypnotically induced analgesia: How effective is hypnosis? *Int J Clin Exp Hypn.* 2000;48(2): 138–53.

96. Gruzelier JH. A review of the impact of hypnosis, relaxation, guided imagery and individual differences on aspects of immunity and health. *Stress.* 2002;5(2): 147–63.

97. Temple R. *Open to Suggestion. The Uses and Abuses of Hypnosis.* (The Aquarian Press, 1989).

98. McMillan CO, Spahr-Schopfer IA, Sikich N, Hartley E and Lerman J. Premedication of children with oral midazolam. *Can J Anaesth.* 1992;39(6):545–50.

99. Malinovsky J-M, Populaire C, Cozian A, Lepage J-Y, Lejus C and Pinaud M. Premedication with midazolam in children. Effect of intranasal, rectal and oral routes on plasma midazolam concentrations. *Anaesthesia.* 1995;50(4):351–4.

100. Cox RG, Nemish U, Ewen A and Crowe MJ. Evidence-based clinical update: does premedication with oral midazolam lead to improved behavioural outcomes in children. *Can J Anesth.* 2006;53(12): 1213–19.

101. Lyseng-Williamson KA. Midazolam oral solution (Ozalin®): a profile of its use for

procedural sedation or premedication before anaesthesia in children. *Drugs Ther Perspect.* [Internet]. 2019;35(6):255–62. Available from https://doi.org/10.1007/s40267-019-00629-5.

102. Moon YE. Paradoxical reaction to midazolam in children. *Korean J Anesthesiol.* 2013;65(1):2–3.

103. Basker S, Singh G and Jacob R. Clonidine in paediatrics – a review. *Indian J Anaesth.* 2009;53:270–80.

104. Gopalakrishnan S and Tobias JD. Premedication: is clonidine the answer? *Saudi J Anaesth.* 2012;6(1):1–4.

105. Kaur M and Singh P. Current role of dexmedetomidine in clinical anesthesia and intensive care. *Anesth Essays Res.* 2011;5(2):128.

106. Scott-Warren VL and Sebastian J. Dexmedetomidine: its use in intensive care medicine and anaesthesia. *BJA Educ.* 2016;16(7):242–6.

107. Mahmoud M and Mason KP. Dexmedetomidine: review, update, and future considerations of paediatric perioperative and periprocedural applications and limitations. *Br J Anaesth.* [Internet]. 2015;115(2):171–82. Available from http://dx.doi.org/10.1093/bja/aev226.

108. Weerink MAS, Struys MMRF, Hannivoort LN, Barends CRM, Absalom AR and Colin P. Clinical pharmacokinetics and pharmacodynamics of dexmedetomidine. *Clin Pharmacokinet.* 2017;56(8):893–913.

109. Peng K, Wu SR, Ji FH and Li J. Premedication with dexmedetomidine in pediatric patients: a systematic review and meta-analysis. *Clinics.* 2014;69(11):777–86.

110. Mion G and Villevieille T. Ketamine pharmacology: an update (Pharmacodynamics and molecular aspects, recent findings). *CNS Neurosci Ther.* 2013;19(6):370–80.

111. Pai A and Heining M. Ketamine. *Contin Educ Anaesthesia. Crit Care Pain.* 2007;7(2):59–63.

112. Howell TK, Smith S, Rushman S and Walker RWM. A comparison of oral transmucosal fentanyl and oral midazolam for premedication in children. *Pediatr Anesth.* 2000;10(6):697.

113. Moore PA, Cuddy MA, Magera JA, Caputo AC, Chen AH and Wilkinson LA. Oral transmucosal fentanyl pretreatment for outpatient general anesthesia. *Anesth Prog.* 2000;47(2):29–34.

114. Ellen McCann M and Kain ZN. The management of preoperative anxiety in children: An update. *Anesth Analg.* 2001;93(1):98–105.

115. Lundeberg S and Roelofse JA. Aspects of pharmacokinetics and pharmacodynamics of sufentanil in pediatric practice. *Paediatr Anaesth.* 2011;21(3):274–9.

116. Zedie N, Amory DW, Wagner BKJ and O'Hara DA. Comparison of intranasal midazolam and sufentanil premedication in pediatric outpatients. *Clin Pharmacol Ther.* 1996;59(3):341–8.

117. Fantacci C, Fabrizio GC, Ferrara P, Franceschi F and Chiaretti A. Intranasal drug administration for procedural sedation in children admitted to pediatric Emergency Room. *Eur Rev Med Pharmacol Sci.* 2018;22(1):217–22.

118. Michienzi K, Mireles R, Wanamaker C, Zemer J and Creighton P. A randomized trial of intra-nasal dexmedetomidine and sufent-anil compared with oral midazolam: A pilot study. *J Pharmacol Clin Toxicol.* [Internet]. 2018;6(4):1114. Available from www.random.

119. World Health Organization. Childhood Autism [Internet]. ICD 10 Version 2016. Available from https://icd.who.int/browse10/2016/en#/F84.1.

120. NICE. Autism spectrum disorder in under 19s: recognition, referral and diagnosis. *Clin Guidel.* [Internet]. 2011:44. Available from www.nice.org.uk/guidance/cg128/resources/autism-spectrum-disorder-in-under-19s-recognition-referral-and-diagnosis-pdf-35109456621253.

121. Sartorius N, Haghir H, Mokhber N, et al. The ICD-10 classification of mental and behavioural disorders. *IACAPAP E-Textb Child Adolesc Ment Health.* 2013;55(1993):135–9.

122. American Psychiatric Association. Diagnostic and Statistical Manual of Mental Disorders (DSM–5). [Internet]. 5th ed., 2013. Available from www .psychiatry.org/psychiatrists/practice/dsm.

123. Hyman SL. New DSM-5 includes changes to autism criteria. AAP News. [Internet]. 2013;4–5. Available from www.aapnews .org.

124. World Health Organization. Hyperkinetic disorder (F90) [Internet]. ICD 10 Version 2016. 2016. Available from http://apps.who .int/classifications/icd10/browse/2015/en#/ F90-F98.

125. Kendall T, Taylor E, Perez A and Taylor C. Attention deficit hyperactivity disorder: diagnosis and management [Internet]. 2008. Available from www.nice.org.uk/ guidance/cg72.

126. NICE. Challenging behaviour and learning disabilities: prevention and interventions for people with learning disabilities whose behaviour challenges [Internet]. 2015. Available from www.nice.org.uk/guidance/ ng11#.

127 Schreibman L. Parent training as a means of facilitating generalization in autistic children. In: Horner RH, Dunlap G and Koegel RL, eds., *Generalization and Maintenance: Life-Style Changes in Applied Settings*. (Baltimore: Brookes, 1988, pp. 21–40).

128. NICE. Antisocial behaviour and conduct disorders in children and young people: recognition and management. 2018 (March 2013). Available from www.nice.org.uk/ guidance/qs59/resources/antisocial-behaviour-and-conduct-disorders-in-children-and-young-people-pdf-2098735573957.

129. I CAN Help enquiry service. Visual Timelines – Practitioners. [Internet]. Available from http://licensing.ican.org.uk/ sites/licensing.ican.org.uk/files/pdfs/ Visual-timelines-factsheet-practitioners .pdf.

130. Lequia J, MacHalicek W and Rispoli MJ. Effects of activity schedules on challenging behavior exhibited in children with autism spectrum disorders: a systematic review.

Res Autism Spectr Disord. 2012;6(1): 480–92.

131. Levy DM. Psychic trauma of operations in children and a note on combat neurosis. *Am J Dis Child.* 1945;1(69):7–25.

132. Kain ZN, Caldwell-Andrews AA, Mayes LC, et al. Trial ARC. Family-centered preparation for surgery improves perioperative outcomes in children. *Anesthesiology.* 2007;106(1):65–74.

133. Fortier MA, Blount RL, Wang S, Mayes LC and Kain ZN. Analysing a family-centred preoperative intervention programme: a dismantling approach. *Br J Anaesth.* 2011;106(5):713–18.

134. Hilly J, Hörlin AL, Kinderf J, et al. Preoperative preparation workshop reduces postoperative maladaptive behavior in children. *Paediatr Anaesth.* 2015;25(10):990–8.

135. Kain ZN, Wang SM, Mayes LC, Caramico LA and Hofstadter MB. Distress during the induction of anesthesia and postoperative behavioral outcomes. *Anesth Analg.* 1999;88(5):1042–7.

136. Tong HJ, Khong J, Ong C, et al. Children's and parents' attitudes towards dentists' appearance, child dental experience and their relationship with dental anxiety. *Eur Arch Paediatr Dent.* 2014;15(6): 377–84.

137. Kumar V, Kamavaram Ellore VP, Mohammed M, Taranath M, Ramagoni NK and Gunjalli G. Children and parent's attitude and preferences of dentist's attire in pediatric dental practice. *Int J Clin Pediatr Dent.* 2015;8(2):102–7.

138. Panda A, Garg I and Bhobe AP. Children's perspective on the dentist's attire. *Int J Paediatr Dent.* 2014;24(2):98–103.

139. Sirin Y, Yucel B, Firat D and Husseinova-Sen S. Assessment of dental fear and anxiety levels in eating disorder patients undergoing minor oral surgery. *J Oral Maxillofac Surg.* 2011;69(8):2078–85.

140. Ravikumar D, Gurunathan D and Karthikeyan S. Children's perception towards pediatric dentist attire: an observation study. *Int J Pedod Rehabil.* 2016;1(2):49.

141. Roohafza H, Pirnia A, Sadeghi M, Toghianifar N, Talaei M and Ashrafi M. Impact of nurses clothing on anxiety of hospitalised children. *J Clin Nurs.* 2009;18(13):1953–9.

142. Festini F, Occhipinti V, Cocco M, et al. Use of non-conventional nurses' attire in a paediatric hospital: A quasi-experimental study. National Center for Biotechnology Information. *J Clin Nurs.* 2009;18(7): 1018–26.

143. Pakseresht M, Hemmatipour A, Gilavand A, Zarea K, Poursangbor T and Sakei-Malehi A. The effect of nurses' uniform color on situational anxiety in the school age inpatients children. *J Res Med Dent Sci.* 2019;7(1):114–20.

144. O'Connor Z. Colour psychology and colour therapy: Caveat emptor. *Color Res Appl.* 2011;36(3):229–34.

145. Boyatzis C. Children's emotional associations with color. *J Genet Psychol.* 1994;155(1):77–85.

146. Hettiarachchi AA and De Silva N. Colour associated emotional and behavioural responses: a study on the associations emerged via imagination. *Built-Environment Sri Lanka.* 2012;11(1):21.

147. Rajae-Joordens RJE and Hanique I. The effect of colored light on arousal and valence in participants primed with colored emotional pictures. Proc Exp Light 2012 [Internet]. 2012;1–4. Available from http:// 2012.experiencinglight.nl/orals.html.

148. Schauss AG. The physiological effect of color on the suppression of human aggression: research on Baker-Miller Pink. *Int J Biosoc Res.* 1985;7(2):55–64.

149. Thabrew H, Stasiak K, Hetrick SE, Wong S, Huss JH and Merry SN. E-Health interventions for anxiety and depression in children and adolescents with long-term physical conditions. *Cochrane Database Syst Rev.* 2018;2018(8).

150. Berne E. *Games People Play: The Basic Handbook of Transactional Analysis* [Internet]. Tantor eBooks, 1996. Available from www.penguinrandomhouse.com/ books/12725/games-people-play-by-eric-berne-md.

151. Wright D and Whalley P. Transactional analysis. *Ind Commer Train.* 1978;10(9): 371–7.

152. Bandler R and Grinder J. *The Structure of Magic: A Book about Language and Therapy.* [Internet]. Science and Behavior Books, 1976. Available from http:// pttpnederland.nl/wp-content/uploads/ 2018/03/The-Structure-of-Magic-Vol-I-by-Richard-Bandler-and-John-Grinder.pdf.

153. Tosey P and Mathison J. Neuro-linguistic programming: its potential for learning and teaching in formal education. Paper presented at the European Conference on Educational Research, University of Hamburg, 17–20 September 2003.

154. Neuro-Linguistic Programming Therapy. Psychol Today [Internet]. Available from www.psychologytoday.com/gb/therapy-types/neuro-linguistic-programming-therapy.

155. British Association of Play Therapists [Internet]. Available from www.bapt.info/ play-therapy/info-professionals-employers.

156. Montgomery GH, David D, Winkel G, Silverstein JH and Bovbjerg DH. The effectiveness of adjunctive hypnosis with surgical patients: A meta-analysis. *Anesth Analg.* 2002;94(6):1639–45.

157. Calipel S, Lucas-Polomeni MM, Wodey E and Ecoffey C. Premedication in children: hypnosis versus midazolam. *Paediatr Anaesth.* 2005;15(4):275–81.

158. O'Byrne KK, Peterson L and Saldana L. Survey of pediatric hospitals' preparation programs: evidence of the impact of health psychology research. *Heal Psychol.* 1997;16:147–54.

159. Kain ZN, Caldwell-Andrews A and Wang SM. Psychological preparation of the parent and pediatric surgical patient. *Anesthesiol Clin N Am.* 2002;20(1): 29–44.

160. Kain ZN, Caldwell-Andrews AA, Mayes LC, et al. Family-centered preparation for surgery improves perioperative outcomes in children: a randomized controlled trial. *Anesthesiology.* 2007;106(1):65–74.

161. Kain ZN, Mayes LC and Caramico LA. Preoperative preparation in children: a

cross-sectional study. *J Clin Anesth.* 1996;8(6):508–14.

162. Kain ZN, Fortier MA, Chorney JM and Mayes L. Web-based tailored intervention for preparation of parents and children for outpatient surgery (WebTIPS): development. *Anesth Analg.* 2015;120(4): 905–6.

163. Chow CHT, Van Lieshout RJ, Schmidt LA, Dobson KG and Buckley N. Systematic review: audiovisual interventions for reducing preoperative anxiety in children undergoing elective surgery. *J Pediatr Psychol.* 2016;41(2):182–203.

164. Batuman A, Gulec E, Turktan M, Gunes Y and Ozcengiz D. Preoperative informational video reduces preoperative anxiety and postoperative negative behavioral changes in children. *Minerva Anesthesiol.* 2016;82(5):534–42.

165. Chow CHT, Wan S, Pope E, et al. Audiovisual interventions for parental preoperative anxiety: a systematic review and meta-analysis. *Heal Psychol.* 2018;37(8):746–58.

166. Hatipoglu Z, Gulec E, Lafli D and Ozcengiz D. Effects of auditory and audiovisual presentations on anxiety and behavioral changes in children undergoing elective surgery. *Niger J Clin Pract.* 2018;21(6): 788–94.

167. Eijlers R, Utens EMWJ, Staals LM, et al. Systematic review and meta-analysis of virtual reality in pediatrics: effects on pain and anxiety. *Anesth Analg.* 2019;129 (5):1344–53.

168. Castellano-Tejedor C and Cencerrado A. Augmented reality: an emerging field in pediatric psycho-oncology requiring research. *Adv Mod Oncol Res.* 2019;4(6): 4–7.

169. XPLORO app [Internet]. Available from https://xploro.health.

170. Little Journey [Internet]. Available from https://littlesparkshospital.com.

171. Bray L, Sharpe A, Gichuru PK, Fortune P-M, Blake L and Appleton V. The acceptability and impact of the Xploro digital therapeutic (DTx) platform to inform and prepare children for planned procedures in hospital: a before-after evaluation study. *J Med Internet Res.* 2020;22(8):e17367.

172. Liguori S, Stacchini M, Ciofi D, Olivini N, Bisogni S and Festini F. Effectiveness of an app for reducing preoperative anxiety in children: a randomized clinical trial. *JAMA Pediatr.* 2016;170(8):1–6.

Index